Medical Transcription

FOR

DUMMIES®

by Anne Martinez

WILEY

John Wiley & Sons, Inc.

Medical Transcription For Dummies®

Published by
John Wiley & Sons, Inc.
111 River St.
Hoboken, NJ 07030-5774
www.wiley.com

WILEY

About the Author

Anne Martinez and medical transcription met for the first time in 2005. She had no idea what she was getting in to. Desiring a little "regular work" to round out her self-employment income, she took to the Internet and began researching work-at-home jobs. Medical transcription seemed a perfect match for her love of language and interest in all things medical. Her first step was to look for an introductory how-to book, but there wasn't one. She determined on the spot that she would write it; first, though, on to becoming a medical transcriptionist!

In 2006, after about a year of intense studying at home, Anne graduated from the M-TEC online medical transcription program. Soon thereafter, she was employed full time (despite her original intention to work part time) and garnering the benefits of health insurance she didn't have to pay for entirely herself, a steady income, and actual paid vacation days! She later switched to a part-time independent contractor position to gain a more flexible schedule and take advantage of additional opportunities.

During her time as an MT, Anne transcribed many, many medical reports for hospitals and physician groups, including history and physical exams, discharge summaries, operative reports, consultations, office notes, and an amazing variety of diagnostic procedures.

She's currently wrapped up in writing projects and managing her successful website, GoCertify (www.gocertify.com), so she's put her MT career on hold. However, it stands ready in the wings, waiting for her return should the need arise.

Dedication

To all the hockey players I've ever played with or against, especially the teams I've been honored to be part of: May your skates always be sharp, the ice hard, and the Zamboni working.

P.S. May your medical records contain only routine office notes.

Author's Acknowledgments

A book is rarely the fruit of a single author, and this one is no different. Many people participated in shaping it and packing it with the most relevant and accessible information possible. My first shout-out goes to Patty Urban, my go-to resource for everything MT since practically day one of my MT career and the natural pick to serve as technical editor of *Medical Transcription For Dummies.*

To Ann Morgan and the other MTs who hang out at the Medical Transcription Networking Corner on Facebook, thank you for sharing your experiences and opinions on all things MT. Carol Butler, Cindy Leach, and Debi Shope made time to contribute thoughtful MT wisdom and advice despite intensely busy schedules.

Others who were instrumental to the creation of this book include Lindsay Lefevere, who gave me the chance to write the book I've been thinking about since I signed up for my first MT course, and Matt Wagner, without whom I never would have met Lindsay. Elizabeth Kuball, project editor extraordinaire, dedicated her time and expertise to make sure this book became the best it could be. Many thanks also to Steve Elliot, who once again pointed me in the right direction when I told him there was a book I wanted to write. Extra kudos to Sara Devine, for relentlessly tracking down permissions and helping keep the rest of my work life running while I focused on this book.

Special thanks to Dan McGovern for his support, encouragement, and friendship that helped carry this book and its author through an onslaught of deadlines, and to my teenage children, Evan and Rebecca, who basically surrendered me to this process and largely took care of themselves for the duration.

Publisher's Acknowledgments

We're proud of this book; please send us your comments at http://dummies.custhelp.com. For other comments, please contact our Customer Care Department within the U.S. at 877-762-2974, outside the U.S. at 317-572-3993, or fax 317-572-4002.

Some of the people who helped bring this book to market include the following:

Acquisitions and Editorial

Project Editor: Elizabeth Kuball

Executive Editor: Lindsay Sandman Lefevere

Copy Editor: Elizabeth Kuball

Assistant Editor: David Lutton

Editorial Program Coordinator: Joe Niesen

Technical Editor: Patricia Urban

Senior Editorial Manager: Jennifer Ehrlich

Editorial Manager: Elizabeth Kuball

Editorial Assistant: Rachelle Amick, Alexa Koschier

Cover Photos: © Feng Yu / iStockphoto.com

Cartoons: Rich Tennant (www.the5thwave.com)

Composition Services

Project Coordinator: Patrick Redmond

Layout and Graphics: Melanie Habig, Jennifer Henry, Andrea Hornberger

Proofreaders: Joni Heredia, Jessica Kramer

Indexer: Steve Rath

Publishing and Editorial for Consumer Dummies

    Kathleen Nebenhaus, Vice President and Executive Publisher

    Kristin Ferguson-Wagstaffe, Product Development Director

    Ensley Eikenburg, Associate Publisher, Travel

    Kelly Regan, Editorial Director, Travel

Publishing for Technology Dummies

    Andy Cummings, Vice President and Publisher

Composition Services

    Debbie Stailey, Director of Composition Services

Contents at a Glance

Table of Contents

Introduction

. . . .

You've probably heard that medical transcription is a flexible career that you can do from home. Perhaps you're attracted to the idea of being part of the drama and intimate details of medical care, and medical transcription sounds like it would be very interesting work. Maybe you just want something, anything, you can do from home to earn a buck, and you're wondering if medical transcription could be it.

Despite what some advertisements might lead you to believe, it's not true that anyone willing to take a course can become a medical transcriptionist (MT) and earn big bucks working from home. It *is* true that it's interesting, challenging, and often flexible work. Many MTs do work from home. You can prepare for and launch an MT career without ever stepping out your front door, if you want to. For some people, it's a great career option, but it's not the right choice for everyone.

About This Book

This isn't a textbook about how to become an MT. You don't need to read it cover to cover or even in order. Dip into the part you need, when you need it. Come back later and dip into a different section when you need that. Consider this a quick study guide, reusable reference, and career companion.

There's a lot of information, and even more misinformation, available about working as a medical transcriptionist. This book is here to help you sort fact from fiction, so you can decide if you want to become an MT, and if so, how to go about it. It's also designed to stand beside you and answer the questions that most commonly pop up after you get on the job.

Conventions Used in This Book

I don't use many conventions in this book, but I do use a few:

✔ When I define a new term, I *italicize* it. You can find the definition nearby (often in parentheses).

✔ I use `monofont` for web and e-mail addresses. ***Note:*** When this book was printed, some web addresses may have needed to break across two lines of text. If that happened, rest assured that we haven't added extra characters (such as hyphens) to indicate the break. So, when using one of these web addresses, just type in exactly what you see in this book, pretending as though the line break doesn't exist.

What You're Not to Read

The shaded boxes that appear here and there are sidebars. They include extra information that's interesting or fun. The material in them isn't essential to understanding the topic at hand, and you can bypass them without missing out on key concepts.

The Technical Stuff icon identifies extras included for people who like to know the details behind things. If you're not one of them, it's okay to zip right past.

Foolish Assumptions

I figure you've probably picked up this book for one of the following reasons:

✔ You're thinking about becoming an MT and you want to know what the job entails and how to get started.

✔ You're already an MT student and you picked up this book to help you get off to a flying start.

✔ You're a working MT who's as obsessed with learning and growing as you've always been.

I also assume that you want to get straight to business and not waste time lollygagging around.

How This Book Is Organized

This book is broken into parts that parallel the journey to an MT career. It starts at the beginning with career exploration and moves on to identifying and mastering practical skills and then to landing and managing an MT job. The final part provides reference materials you can use to help you on the job.

Every chapter in *Medical Transcription For Dummies* is designed to be entirely self-contained. You can go through them in order or jump straight to whatever you need at the moment. This is one time when you can have something both ways.

Part 1: So, You Want to Be a Medical Transcriptionist

Before diving into a career in medical transcription, you'll want to know exactly what's involved and what to expect. This part will give you the basis to decide if medical transcription is a realistic career option for you, and if so, how to get off to a running start. It starts with an inside look at what MTs do on a daily basis and what it really takes to break into the field. You'll also survey the types of places MTs work and how much you can expect to earn. One of the most crucial foundations to a successful MT launch is getting the right training. This part identifies what that should include so you don't spend good money on bad training.

Part II: Getting the Job Done: Medical Transcriptionist How-To

This is where you'll meet and build the technical skills that lie at the heart of a successful medical transcription career. You can put yourself through medical terminology boot camp and study up on the mechanics of formatting medical reports following accepted standards. There's also a chapter packed with tips for deciphering difficult dictation and tricks for coping with mumbly mouthed dictators. In medical transcription, time is (your) money. The chapters on effective referencing and speed-boosting techniques will help you lay in the skills so you can be fast and accurate.

Part III: Looking At the Types of Reports You'll Transcribe

This part takes you on an in-depth tour of individual reports and how to transcribe them. Each member of the "Big Four" family of reports gets its own detailed chapter. You also step through another half-dozen report types you're likely to encounter.

Part IV: Employment Matters: Landing and Managing a Medical Transcriptionist Job

MT skills are useful only if you can put them to work! This part offers tips and advice to help you choose and land your first MT job — and the one after that. There's a chapter explaining the technical details of outfitting a home office. If you opt to work as an independent contractor (IC), you'll want to read the chapter on financial matters, for sure.

Part V: The Part of Tens

If you're a fan of top ten lists, this is the part for you. It includes ten factors that contribute to MT success, busts ten common myths about medical transcription work, and introduces you to ten online resources that stand head and shoulders above the rest.

Part VI: Appendixes

Good references are among an MT's best allies. The glossary, transcription examples, and sample reports in this part are here for you to turn to when you need a little help. They don't eradicate the need for dedicated reference books, but they do provide a unique cross-section of material that zeroes in on the items experience shows you're most likely to need.

Icons Used in This Book

As you go through this book, you'll see the following cute little icons in the margins. Here's what they mean:

The Tip icon points out a handy technique or shortcut that can save you time or help you avoid frustration down the road.

When you see the Remember icon, it's pointing out a key concept you'll want to file away in your brain for future use.

The Warning icon alerts you to potential pitfalls and things that can cause serious trouble. When you see it, pay extra-careful attention to the text nearby.

The Technical Stuff icon points out technical tidbits that are interesting but not absolutely necessary to understanding the topic at hand. If you want all the details you can get, read them. If you want just the basics, skip them.

Where to Go from Here

By all means, jump into this book anywhere you'd like. If you're in an exploratory phase, Chapter 1 is the obvious place to begin, but you may also head on over to the Part of Tens and start by clearing up ten myths about medical transcription. If you want to take a gander at some actual medical reports, Appendix C has you covered.

If you're burning to steep yourself in medical terminology as quickly as possible, the boot camp in Chapter 5 is specifically for you. If difficult dictators have you hog-tied, Chapter 7 will help you decipher what they are (in theory) saying. Working MTs and students near graduation may be particularly interested in the "faster, faster" productivity techniques in Chapter 9.

Thinking about going the independent contractor instead of employee route? Be sure to read Chapter 19 so you can get your financial ducks in a row and keep them there.

You also can read this book in the ordinary, straightforward manner: Start at the beginning and keep going until there are no pages left to turn.

Part I

So, You Want to Be a Medical Transcriptionist

The 5th Wave   By Rich Tennant

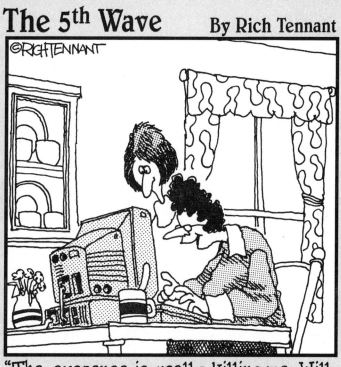

"The suspense is really killing me. Will he administer 4mL or 5mL of lidocaine?"

In this part . . .

Time to cut through the hype and clutter and get to the facts on a medical transcriptionist career. As a medical transcriptionist, you'll make critical contributions to patient care that go far beyond typing fast. This section gives you an inside look at what medical transcriptionists do on a daily basis and the personal traits and professional skills required to get the job done. It also surveys where the jobs are, how much they pay, and how to get the training needed to break into the field.

Chapter 1

Just the Facts

- -

- -

*1*f you're considering a career in medical transcription, there are some things you should know. The very first is that what medical transcriptionists (MTs) actually do all day is a whole lot more interesting and much more difficult than what most people think. Typing fast while listening to someone speak in tongues over headphones is just the tip of the iceberg.

Okay, the dictator isn't really speaking in tongues, but it often sounds like she is, and the iceberg part is completely true. In this chapter, you'll explore the 90 percent of medical transcription that most people never see because it's out of sight, just like the largest part of an iceberg.

If you've heard that a lot of MTs work from home, you are, indeed, well informed. For many MTs, the daily commute is no farther than the walk from their breakfast table to their home office. Some MTs commute to their place of work, just like other employees, although these seem to be dwindling in number.

Medical transcription work has many attributes that attract people looking for a fresh career start. You can train and work from practically anywhere you can get an Internet connection, including your home. Nobody cares what you look like or how old you are; the only thing that matters is whether you can do the job well. Schedules often can be juggled so that you can work around other commitments.

It's not all peaches and cream, however. Medical transcription can be high-stress work, and you aren't likely to get rich doing it. It takes a particular set of personality traits and technical skills to survive and thrive in an MT career. This chapter introduces the world of medical transcription, so that you can decide if you want to become a part of it.

Getting the Skinny on the Medical Transcription Field

A medical transcriptionist's job is to produce the clearest, most accurate healthcare documentation possible — and do it fast. Within the course of a day, a patient who comes into a hospital emergency room and is admitted with appendicitis will generate:

- An emergency room (ER) report
- Probably a CT scan or ultrasound of the abdomen
- A consultation with a gastroenterologist and/or a surgeon
- A complete preoperative history and physical examination
- An operative report detailing the appendectomy
- Potentially periodic progress notes
- A discharge summary when sent home the next day

And all of them require transcription. That's one patient, one hospital, one overnight stay. Multiply that by the number of patients who walk into hospitals each day, seven days a week.

Hospitals aren't the only prodigious producers of medical reports. Physician practices, specialty clinics, alternative health practitioners, managed care organizations, diagnostic facilities, and lots of other places all generate dictation every day.

These are the records that healthcare providers return to time and again when deciding what treatments a patient will receive immediately and in the future. They're also legal documents. They may be used to determine whether someone is eligible to receive disability benefits and how much. In some cases, they'll be pulled out when determining compensation for an injury or death that occurred as the result of someone else's actions.

MT work is interesting, intellectually challenging, and a whole lot harder than people who've never done it can imagine. Many people spend good money on MT training, only to find that they don't like doing medical transcription, and it doesn't like them much either. Other people absolutely love it. The people who love it tend to share certain personality traits. Top among them are

- A love of language and a passion for learning
- The desire and ability to work independently and sometimes under pressure
- A perfectionistic streak that makes attention to tiny details come naturally

Where the jobs are

MTs work in hospitals, physician practices, and other types of facilities. Many MTs are employed by medical transcription service organizations (MTSOs). An MTSO is a service bureau for medical transcription work. Many medical facilities that used to perform transcription in house now outsource it to MTSOs, making them a top source of MT employment.

It's hard to say exactly how many people are currently doing MT work. The Bureau of Labor Statistics (BLS) estimates that nearly 79,000 MTs were on employer payrolls in 2010. There are actually a lot more than that, because BLS figures don't include self-employed MTs, of which there are many. Self-employed MTs work as independent contractors (ICs), providing transcription services to one or more transcription clients.

How much they pay

MT earnings are hard to pin down for similar reasons: A lot of people aren't counted. The BLS figures put the 2011 average annual wage for MTs across all industries at $34,050 and the hourly wage at $16.37. MTs working for medical and diagnostic laboratories or for general hospitals earn more than the average. Employees of business support services earn a bit less.

The BLS has the largest pool of pay data, but because it doesn't include self-employed MTs, it's a very incomplete picture. Figures available through Salary.com are more current, though less extensive. As of May 2012, Salary.com reported the average MT base salary to be $38,695.

Although MT pay is reported using hourly and annual figures, it's usually calculated based on production. MTs typically earn a fixed amount for each line they transcribe. An MT making 8 cpl (cents per line) would earn $100 for transcribing 1250 lines ($1250 \times 0.08 = \$100$).

The number of lines a transcriptionist produces in any given day is affected by many factors. Some MTs have a target number of lines and work until they reach it; others work a set number of hours and transcribe as many lines as they can within that time. If you're quick and have good dictation to work with, you can really crank out the reports and rack up your line count. On the downside, a string of really terrible dictators can slow your production and, thus, your earnings to a virtual standstill and make you feel like pulling your hair out.

To really dig into the details of MT job options and pay, head to Chapter 3.

What it takes to break in

You don't need a license or certification to work as an MT, but formal training is an absolute must. Without it, no one will hire you. Even if you could miraculously wrangle your way in the door, to survive on the job, you're going to need to tune up skills you already have and learn entirely new ones. There are two really good places to get MT training:

- **Community colleges:** Community college programs come with the benefits of classmates, a fixed schedule to keep you on track, and face-to-face interaction with your instructors.

- **Online MT schools:** Online programs free you to study on your own schedule, without leaving home. Online courses can be a great option for people with the self-discipline to study regularly and stay on track.

Either type of training will provide you all the skills needed to get out of the starting gate.

The quality of MT training programs varies greatly, and choosing a bad one can be an expensive and frustrating mistake. Chapter 4 provides additional information to help you choose wisely.

Studying to become an MT is guaranteed to be interesting, but it won't be as quick as some advertisements may lead you to believe. Fast learners with plenty of time to devote to studying can complete an MT training program in about nine months. Most students require a bit longer. If you'll be fitting studying in around a busy family life and/or a job, plan on a year or even two.

MT employers expect even new MTs to arrive ready to hit the ground running, although you'll continue to learn on the job. Absorb and practice as much as you possibly can while a student — you'll be really glad you did later. While you're at it, earn the highest GPA you possibly can. The higher your GPA, the easier it will be for you to land your first MT job.

Before you plunk down tuition and devote yourself to MT training (or decide not to), be sure to read Chapter 22. There's quite a bit of MT fiction floating around, and Chapter 22 tackles it head-on.

Looking at What Goes into Good Transcription

A lot more goes into producing the neat, clear medical reports we all prefer to have in our health records than is apparent by reading them. MTs remove ambiguities, clean up jargon, and catch inadvertent errors that could prove catastrophic if they slipped by unnoticed. They take often messy input and turn it into a report that's clear to everyone who reads it going forward, not just the person who originally dictated it. And they have to do it quickly, or else it's cheerio, old chap — good luck in your next career!

To accomplish these feats, MTs apply skills that go far beyond listening well and typing fast. Truly understanding the language of medicine ranks at the top. It's not just a matter of memorization, thank goodness! Memorizing even a fraction of the 120,000-plus terms in a standard 2,000-page medical dictionary would take a very, very long time. MTs don't have to do that, because most medical terms are built from a set of reusable parts, combined and recombined to generate new meanings. MTs know the parts and how they work together. That makes the meaning of even unfamiliar terms instantly recognizable, and conveniently also possible to spell and pronounce. Without this knowledge, recognizing a term like *choledocholithotomy* the first time you heard it would be nearly impossible; with it, it's a piece of cake. Chapter 5 provides a crash course on exactly how to do this.

Not all core MT skills are as fun as mastering medical lingo, but they're necessary nonetheless. Not coincidentally, the better you are at them, the more successful your MT career will be. A solid MT

- ✔ Has a well-stocked arsenal of tips and tricks for deciphering difficult dictators, whether they be mumblers, speed talkers, or people who haven't mastered speaking English to the same degree that they've mastered practicing medicine

- ✔ Is an expert on the nuances of formatting, punctuating, and capitalizing every aspect of medical reports according to industry standards

- ✔ Knows how to quickly sleuth out details to confirm, rule out, or pin down a slippery word, phrase, medication dosage, facility name, or anything else

- ✔ Is well versed in MT productivity tools and techniques, so they can transcribe as quickly and efficiently as possible

The MT uses all these skills to do one, not-so-simple thing: transcribe a healthcare provider's spoken words into a neat, clear, and accurate medical report.

Anticipating What You'll Transcribe

A lot of MT work involves transcribing a core set of reports nicknamed the Big Four. They're so central that this book dedicates a chapter to each of them. They are

> ✔ History and Physical examinations (H&P; Chapter 10)
>
> ✔ Consultations (Chapter 11)
>
> ✔ Operative reports (Chapter 12)
>
> ✔ Discharge and death summaries (Chapter 13)

The Big Four make up a large share of MT work, but they're accompanied by a huge constellation of other report types. For starters, an incredible variety of diagnostic procedures is used to probe the human body and pinpoint what's gone awry, ranging from EEGs to echocardiograms and Doppler ultrasounds, to overnight sleep studies where the patient is wired up to more sensors than a crash-test dummy and every breath recorded and analyzed. All these diagnostic studies generate reports that need to be transcribed.

Another large batch of transcription work arrives in the form of routine office notes and progress reports. They come from checking up on Mr. Smith's diabetes, diagnosing Mrs. Jones's pregnancy with twins, and following up on Grandpa Bill's long list of age-related ailments. These give you a true cross-section of the human condition and make you appreciate your own health.

MTs also transcribe special-purpose reports, such as psychiatric assessments, autopsy reports, and independent medical evaluations (IMEs), among others.

Making a Career of Medical Transcription

Somewhere between deciding you're about ready to hit the job market and starting to polish up your résumé, you're going to have to make a few key decisions, among them:

> ✔ **What type of medical transcription do you want to do?** Some MTs are eager to dive in to a fast-paced acute care transcription environment; others find working for a small physician group or clinic more attractive. Becoming a specialist in a field like diagnostic radiology is an option, though it's one that's not widely available to entry-level MTs.
>
> ✔ **Do you want to work as an independent contractor or as an employee?** MTs can find work as either an employee or as an IC. Both are very common, but they're quite different propositions. The first is an employer-employee relationship; the other, a business-to-business (B2B) relationship. Each has pros and cons to consider:

- Employees are under the direct control of an employer. They have to do what the employer dictates, including working particular hours, working extra hours, or using specific methods. It's the kind of arrangement that anyone who's ever held even a part-time job is familiar with.

- Independent contractors, on the other hand, are self-employed. An IC is essentially running a business providing MT services. ICs have greater control over their work schedule and workload. They do, however, have to take on more taxes and don't get to take advantage of employer-provided benefits. There's a lot more to the IC picture, so if it's on your list of possibilities, check out Chapter 19 for a detailed look at the financial ins and outs of working as an IC.

Once you start job shopping, you'll quickly discover that one-stop job boards like CareerBuilder (`www.careerbuilder.com`) and Monster (`www.monster.com`) contain a bountiful supply of MT openings. Unfortunately, nearly all of them seek applicants with at least two years of experience, something that newly graduated MTs just don't have. Fortunately, there are better places to look first anyway. In fact, your first (or your next) MT job may be as nearby as your training school's list of connections. That's one of the best places to start a fresh job search. Online MT communities and professional relationships are top resources, too. As with any other career, there's no guarantee there will be a slew of employers waiting for you with open arms the minute you graduate. Some new graduates find employment right away; others really have to work at it.

MT employers routinely require applicants to pass a skills test as part of the application process. Just when you thought you were done with those pesky things, too! Pre-employment tests are an easy way for employers to weed out people who think they're qualified but really aren't. Take it as a piece of job security and further evidence that MT work is much more skilled than it appears on the surface. Your first test probably will be a little nerve-wracking, but if you know your stuff, you'll pass with flying colors.

Once you're on the job, you'll discover something else about MT work that most people don't know: At times, it's really quite entertaining. When a doctor says something like "The patient came to see me today because she wants to get pregnant," or "He denies a foul odor to his diarrhea," how can you help but laugh?

MTs learn something new each and every day. It may be an interesting term, like *furuncle,* or running across HELLP syndrome or Christmas disease for the first time.

Medicine and technology are inextricably intertwined, and both evolve at an astounding rate. As an MT, you'll need to evolve with them. It helps to be a passionate learner, as most MTs are.

Some of the largest changes right now involve the widely trumpeted arrival of speech recognition technology (SRT) and the federally mandated move to electronic health records (EHRs). Some people think these two things spell doom for the medical transcription field. Those are primarily the same people who focus on the top 10 percent of an iceberg and completely ignore the other 90 percent.

For example, speech recognition has come a long way, but MTs who clean up after it call it "speech wreck" for a reason. Only a computer can take "This is a 5-foot 6, 145-pound male" and turn it into "This is a 5-foot, 6,145-pound male," or mindlessly record that a male patient underwent a radical hysterectomy. This is the kind of stuff that's going to replace medical transcriptionists? What a terrifying prospect from the patient's perspective! Medical malpractice attorneys and insurance providers must find it horrifying as well.

These particular boo-boos never made it into patient records, because MTs caught and corrected them first. But things like them occur all the time. Sometimes as many as 40 to 50 in a two-minute dictation. I couldn't find a single MT who has ever seen an error-free SRT report. Not one, ever. Obviously, "speech wreck" won't be replacing MTs any time soon. In fact, in some ways, it provides job security.

EHR is not likely to eliminate the need for MTs either. Healthcare providers need a way to include free-form opinions and discussion. Dictation provides it, and MTs are integral to making dictation work.

Things like new technologies and healthcare legislation impact how an MT carries out her job. The underlying mission, however, remains the same: to produce the most clear and accurate healthcare documentation possible, and do it fast! If you think that's something you could learn to do, and want to do, then an MT career may be in your future. This book is here to help you decide if you and medical transcription are a good match. If the answer turns out to be yes, it's also here to help you make it happen.

Chapter 2

The What, How, Who, and Why of Medical Transcription

- -

In This Chapter

▶ Surveying the field of medical transcription

▶ Getting the lowdown on how medical records are transcribed

▶ Considering if you have what it takes to be a successful medical transcriptionist

▶ Identifying the benefits of working as a medical transcriptionist

- -

*Y*ou may have seen ads or attended a seminar that promised you can be trained as a medical transcriptionist and work from home (in your pajamas if you like) within weeks. Surely you can become a medical transcriptionist with minimal training — after all, it's just typing what somebody says, right? Actually, no. Medical transcriptionists (MTs for short) create records and reports that are used to make critical decisions about patients' healthcare. They're experts in medical language, driven to pursue perfection, and able to apply critical thinking and research skills deftly and quickly.

Medical transcription is a lot more complex and quite a bit more challenging than many people expect. In this chapter, I explain how medical transcriptionists transform words spoken by a medical professional into a formal medical record. You find out what goes on between the moment the words leave a dictator's lips and the time it becomes a permanent part of a patient's medical record. You explore the skills and personality traits that contribute to a successful and enjoyable medical transcription career and complete a short self-assessment to determine if you and medical transcription are a good match. Finally, I fill you in on the advantages of a career in medical transcription.

What Medical Transcriptionists Do

Medical transcriptionists are supposed to produce the most accurate and clear healthcare documentation possible, often on very tight deadlines. And they must do so even if the physician has a heavy accent or dictates while gulping down dinner, and even if loud conversations, a wailing baby, or medical alarms are going off in the background.

Under such conditions, the MT must reconcile the duty to transcribe verbatim (exactly what the doctor says word for word) with the responsibility to produce high-quality reports, and juggle both of those tasks with the reality of a job that usually pays on production: The faster you go, the more you earn.

If the MT introduces a mistake into a patient's medical record, such as mistyping a medication name or dosage, the results can be serious — even deadly. If the dictator makes a mistake and the MT catches it, the MT averts a potential disaster for that patient.

When you understand the true challenges and responsibilities associated with being an MT, the job can quickly go from easy to intimidating. Yet these same challenges and responsibilities make the job interesting and rewarding.

Officially: It's about documentation

The job of a medical transcriptionist is to convert spoken medical information into formal medical records. The dictations cover everything from routine healthcare to life-threatening emergencies. The collection of the resulting documents becomes the patient's medical history. Health professionals rely on them when assessing a patient's past care, current status, and future needs.

Officially speaking, there are two formal, published descriptions of what functions a medical transcriptionist performs. The job description the U.S. Department of Labor uses is pretty slim:

> Transcribe medical reports recorded by physicians and other healthcare practitioners using various electronic devices, covering office visits, emergency room visits, diagnostic imaging studies, operations, chart reviews, and final summaries. Transcribe dictated reports and translate abbreviations into fully understandable form. Edit as necessary and return reports in either printed or electronic form for review and signature, or correction.

Don't hold the brevity of this against the Department of Labor writers, though; they only get a single a paragraph to summarize an entire profession.

The second formal medical transcription job description is published by the Association for Healthcare Documentation Integrity (AHDI). This job description (which is too long and detailed to reproduce here) organizes the MT profession into three career levels and delves into the expected knowledge and job functions of each. It's updated from time to time; the current version is available on the AHDI website (www.ahdionline.org).

These official descriptions are deliberately succinct, and that means they summarize in generalities at the expense of particulars. They don't have room, for example, to mention that a lot of the communication between healthcare providers and, thus, a lot of work done by transcriptionists revolves around a set of reports dubbed the "Big Four":

✔ **History and Physical Examination (H&P):** The standard medical intake report describing who you are and what your problem is. These reports are dictated in new-patient office visits and acute-care facilities.

✔ **Consultation:** What the specialist says before he sends the bill.

✔ **Operative Report:** What happened under the knife.

✔ **Discharge Summary:** How it all worked out in the end.

Although the Big Four make the biggest splash, there is a virtually endless variety of reports to transcribe. Which ones a particular MT encounters on a regular basis depends on where he works. Other common report types include the following:

✔ **Office/clinic note:** Summary of an office visit, often just a paragraph or two per patient and often dictated in a series as each patient is seen.

✔ **Independent medical evaluation (IME):** An in-depth assessment of past treatment and current condition, used to determine eligibility for workers' compensation and insurance benefits, as evidence in personal injury or negligence lawsuits, and in other legal proceedings. As you may expect from any document related to potential litigation, these reports can go on for pages. They're also often quite interesting.

✔ **Diagnostic report:** Findings on X-rays, ultrasounds, CT scans, MRIs, echocardiograms, sleep studies, and other diagnostic procedures. They're generally short and quantitative.

✔ **Emergency room reports, physical therapy evaluations, psychiatric assessments, birth and death summaries, and more.**

MTs take steps to enhance the clarity of reports as they transcribe them, including

✔ Expanding medical acronyms, many of which can have different meanings depending on context

✔ Applying rules of English grammar and punctuation, regardless of whether the dictator follows them

✔ Formatting the reports following standard guidelines and facility-specific rules

✔ Tracking down and flagging potential errors

In addition to transcribing spoken dictation, MTs are increasingly handed the task of proofreading, editing, and correcting medical documents created using speech recognition technology (SRT). MTs also must understand and comply with patient privacy and confidentiality guidelines, including the federal HIPAA regulations that define national standards for the management and protection of health information.

These activities comprise the public face of MT work. They're the aspects most apparent to those on the outside looking in.

Unofficially: Critical contributions to patient care

The overriding mission of an MT is to produce a medical record that is clear and accurate, even if the original source of information is not. It requires employing personal judgment and no small amount of patience and determination. If all medical dictators spoke clearly, used good dictation equipment in proper working order, clearly enunciated any jargon they use, and never made mistakes, medical transcription would be largely a matter of typing fast and referencing accurately. Modern computer programs could do it virtually unaided. However, the real world is rarely neat and tidy, and neither is dictation.

MTs clean up after dictators who are hampered by their equipment or surroundings, fatigued, or just plain bad communicators. They do it carefully, thoroughly, and often under tight deadlines. MTs apply knowledge of medical terminology, surgical procedures, lab tests, medications, and human anatomy and physiology to correctly transcribe often complex medical encounters. They detect and correct mistakes. An MT is sometimes the difference maker between a barely legible medical record and crystal clear one.

A rose by any other name: Alternate job titles

In an effort to reflect the changing responsibilities and variety of important roles medical transcriptionists fill, alternative job titles sometimes are used:

✔ Clinical documentation specialist

✔ Medical language specialist (MLS)

✔ Healthcare documentation specialist

✔ Healthcare documentation practitioner

✔ Health information professional

✔ Medical speech recognition editor

Medical transcriptionist (MT) is still the most widely used job title, though.

The fellow human being whose care is being recorded is the ultimate beneficiary of an MT's efforts, but not the only one. Many dictators recognize this and appreciate the extra layer of support and even safety MTs provide. High-quality healthcare documentation is critical to the survival of healthcare facilities, too. It's central to their ability to

✔ Increase patient safety

✔ Comply with extensive state and federal regulations

✔ Reduce risk exposure and potentially lower liability costs from lawsuits

✔ Obtain payment from health-insurance providers, which want to know exactly what treatment a patient has received and from who before coughing up a dime

How Medical Transcription Works

Back in the day (sometime between the Stone Age and the dawn of the Internet), dictation was done into tape recorders or over the phone (to a bigger tape recorder). Transcriptionists would then play back the tapes through headphones, using transcription equipment that allowed them to start, stop, fast-forward, and rewind the tape with a foot pedal, and type what they heard using IBM Selectric typewriters. They were masters of wielding Wite-Out and typewriter correction tape.

Making corrections always has been and always will be part of an MT's tasks. Dictators often don't dictate in a straight line from beginning to end, which can make producing a coherent technical report challenging. Even when they are speaking clearly and not with a mouthful of crackers, they tend to say something, then back up and change it, resume where they previously left off, pause and ask the transcriptionist to insert a new paragraph in the middle of the report, correct a medication dose they dictated earlier, get interrupted, forget what they already said and repeat it, and so forth. They simply don't go straight from point A to point B.

Although the tools have changed, the transcription process remains largely the same. Dictation is done into digital recorders or over the phone (to a bigger digital recorder). Transcriptionists then play back the recording through headphones, using a foot pedal or keyboard controls that allow them to start, stop, fast-forward, and rewind the recording, and perhaps most important, replay it very slowly. They type what they hear into a computer. They're masters of macros and keyboard commands that search and replace and insert and delete text, and thank goodness for spell-check. Dictators still often take side trips in the middle of a report, but it's easier to deal with them.

The journey a report travels from patient encounter to permanent medical record goes like this:

1. A patient visits a healthcare professional or undergoes a medical or diagnostic procedure.

2. The care provider uses a voice-recording device to create a verbal record of the encounter or diagnostic results. The dictator may speak into a handheld recorder, use a phone-in system, or dictate directly into a computer terminal.

3. The report is transmitted over a secure connection to a central server, where it is placed in a "pool" and then funneled into a medical transcriptionist's job queue.

4. The medical transcriptionist accesses the voice recording, listens to it, and transcribes it into the required format.

5. The transcribed report may be "put on hold" to undergo a quality assurance (QA) process.

6. The report is transmitted back to the medical facility and becomes a part of the patient's medical record.

When a report arrives back at the originating facility, it's ideally reviewed by the dictator for accuracy, signed, and added to the patient's medical record. Some dictators don't review their transcribed reports, and those are tagged as "dictated but not read" and receive an electronic version of the dictator's signature. Figure 2-1 illustrates the flow of information from dictator to transcriptionist and back again.

Today the vast majority of MTs work from home and access their job queue remotely using a personal computer and an Internet connection or dedicated telephone line.

With increasing frequency, Step 4 incorporates a detour via speech recognition technology (SRT). Instead of an MT listening to a voice file and creating the report, a computer program takes a preliminary whack at it. The text translation and original audio file are forwarded to an MT, who listens to the voice file and compares it to the text translation, editing as needed to produce the final report. In theory, this approach is faster and requires less skill than transcribing without computer intervention. Experienced MTs, however, report otherwise. Despite the advances in SRT, the editing required can be extensive. The MT must listen to the entire voice file to check for misinterpretations or phrases that were dropped entirely. Minor oddities and major errors must be recognized and remedied. At times, the SRT detour results in greater speed and efficiency, but it also can have the opposite effect.

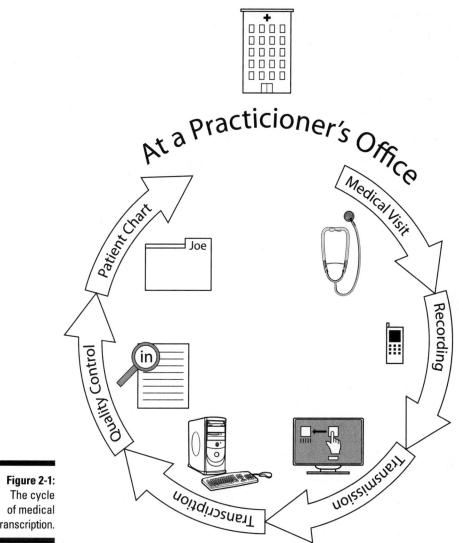

At a Practicioner's Office

Patient Chart

Medical Visit

Quality Control

Recording

Transcription

Transmission

The most satisfied and successful MTs are adaptable and embrace technological change rather than do battle with it. The growing use of SRT is a prime
example. Although SRT won't eliminate the need for traditional transcription
any time soon, many MTs serve as speech recognition editors at least some of
the time.

Who Makes for Good Medical Transcriptionists: The Traits You Need

Working as a medical transcriptionist isn't for everybody. The entry requirements are relatively low when compared to professions that require a college degree or extended apprenticeships and internships, but you'll still have to invest substantial time and money to obtain the training needed to break into the field. You also may have to lay out some cash for equipment and supplies. Before you clear out your schedule and open your wallet, take the time to assess how your personality and skills match up with the demands of the job.

Knowledge of medical terminology and procedures

Medical-speak is virtually a language of its own, and you're going to have to be fluent in it. If you're an avid follower of health issues and a veteran of do-it-yourself Internet self-diagnosis, you already have a head start. If you're already working in a health field, you have an even bigger lead. In either case, however, you'll need to know even more medical lingo to be a successful MT. Although you don't have to memorize every medical procedure, anatomical feature, and surgical implement, you do need to know a lot of them. Otherwise, you'll spend a huge amount of time looking words up, and you'll get extremely frustrated and not earn very much.

If you aren't an expert in medical terminology, don't cancel your MT plans just yet — it's totally learnable with some diligent study. For tips on how medical terms are constructed, turn to Chapter 5 — that'll carry you a long way. Medical terminology is also covered widely and deeply in all MT training courses — it's one of the most enjoyable parts of any MT curriculum.

A love of language and keen interest in the medical field are two things you absolutely must have if you're going to enjoy life as an MT.

English grammar and punctuation skills

MTs add punctuation and fix grievously incorrect grammar in more reports than not. Who dictates punctuation anyway? You may expect people who've graduated from medical school to construct perfect sentences every time, but like the rest of us, they frequently don't. Perhaps it's because there are other things higher on their priority list — little things like accurately describing a patient's neurological symptoms or knee replacement surgery. Nonetheless, medical documentation standards can be absolutely fanatical when it comes to punctuation. There's an entire book dedicated to issues like putting commas and semicolons in the right places and what you should capitalize when transcribing medical documents. Although you won't have to diagram any sentences, you will need better-than-average grammar and punctuation abilities.

Top-notch reference skills

Playing detective is part of an MT's daily duties, and modern MTs are masters of looking things up. Today's MT usually has the benefit of a supply of reference books on hand (either electronic or good old paper and ink) packed with lists of surgical instruments, medical acronyms, brand and generic drug names, and endless other medical minutiae to help fill in the blanks. Barring success there, there's always Google. When a tricky dictation rears its head, the key to cracking the case is knowing where to look and how to do it efficiently. Chapter 8 stands ready to help you.

Keen listening skills

Most people don't listen as well as they think they do. Hearing is the physical reception of sound waves by your ears. Listening is what you do with them. A good listener is able to discern incomplete or mispronounced words and tell the difference between tiny words such as *if* and *of.* A truly skilled listener is automatically alert to context and notices when something doesn't sound quite right, an ability that's essential in medical transcription.

How important are these skills? Consider the medical prefixes *hyper-* and *hypo-.* They sound very similar but have opposite meanings: One means too much and the other means too little. Someone with hypertension has high blood pressure; someone with hypotension has low blood pressure. Getting those the wrong way around could be disastrous — whether or not it's what the dictator actually said.

Ability to work under pressure

Some people thrive under pressure; others wilt. The closer you are to the thrive end of the spectrum, the better off you'll be. As these revealing excerpts from MT job ads show, pressure tolerance isn't just desirable, it's required:

> "must be able to work well under pressure"

> "ability to work under pressure with time constraints"

> "ability to work under pressure with tight deadlines required"

> "ability to work under pressure in a fast-paced environment with time constraints"

The pressure MTs face comes from at least three directions at once:

- ✔ **Reports must be transcribed and returned to the dictator within a specified turnaround time (TAT).** Sometimes it's a matter of medical urgency; other times it's a matter of contractual obligation.

- ✔ **Speed and quality are both important, but they don't always play nicely together.** Taking the time required to ensure quality documentation is often at odds with the pay-per-line nature of most MT compensation. The more lines you transcribe, the greater your paycheck, pushing you to produce reports as quickly as possible. Yet accuracy is of crucial importance, pulling you to slow down and be extra careful. When complex reports or challenging dictators lands in your job queue, which happens frequently, production goes down and stress goes up.

- ✔ **Someone else's fate is at least to some extent in your hands.** Your work performance plays a role in the healthcare another human being receives. Whether you're typing the first report of the day or the twentieth, the pressure is on to make no mistakes.

Even the most independent, stress-resistant MTs want to pull their hair out at times, but those with a resilient personality bounce back quickly. In fact, many MTs pride themselves on their ability to continue unperturbed, no matter what crosses their desks.

Ability to work with little or no supervision

You must be self-motivated, self-disciplined, and comfortable with constantly making judgments on your own if you want to be an MT. Most MT work is home based, which means that the only person with the power to make you get to your desk and stay there is yourself. On the upside, there's no supervisor watching every move you make and no co-workers to distract you with idle chat, but there's also no one nearby to help resolve a difficult dictation. Although you won't be completely incommunicado, most of the time you'll be hunting down references and making judgment calls on your own. Dirty dishes and social invitations from well-meaning friends who don't understand that you're working from home, not sitting at home, will constantly beckon, and you have to muster the resolve to resist their call and keep working.

A perfectionistic streak

Good transcription requires attention to details, details, and even more details. You must be certain that every letter of every phrase you type is 100 percent accurate, down to the last *in* and *on*. When you aren't absolutely certain of a word or phrase, you can't just guestimate — you have to stop and look it up. Nor can you turn in transcriptions with more holes than a kitchen colander or you'll quickly be out of a job. To be a successful MT, you must have a built-in, compelling urge to make things just right and the patience to do it.

Laserlike focus

Maintaining intense concentration for hours at a time, day after day, is one of the most challenging aspects of medical transcription. You must tune out the outside world and home in on every syllable that comes over your headphones, including many that are barely discernible. Every report requires your full concentration. If your thoughts wander even for an instant, you may miss something crucial, or at the very least have to back up the dictation and replay the section you missed.

Don't underestimate the physical stamina required to do medical transcription. Sitting at a computer typing and focusing intently for hours is very tiring and has a way of aggravating existing aches and pains and provoking new ones. Creating an ergonomic workspace, as described in Chapter 20, helps a lot; however, if you already have neck, back, shoulder, wrist, or eye problems, MT work is likely to exacerbate them despite your best ergonomic efforts.

Assessing yourself: Do you have what it takes?

If an MT career sounds great to you so far, read through more of this book before you decide to take the plunge. There are both benefits and drawbacks to working as a medical transcriptionist. Some people dive into an MT career only to discover — after they've invested a lot of time and money in the process — that it doesn't work out at all as they expected, a situation they could've avoided with a little upfront research. Other new MTs quickly grow to love working in medical transcription, enjoy the terminology and patient stories, and get a good laugh when they encounter ridiculous phrases such as *the baby was present at birth.*

The following quiz will help you explore whether you and MT are a good match. Relax — your answers won't be recorded on your permanent record.

Part 1: Your wordsmithing skills

Directions (1–5): Pick the word that properly completes the sentence. (**Hint:** Pay attention to whether it's an adjective, verb, or noun.)

1. I will see her Monday for (follow up / follow-up).

2. Examination of the throat revealed pale (mucus / mucous) membranes.

3. Patient's (affect / effect) was blunted.

4. The umbilical (cord / chord) was clamped and cut.

5. A complete metabolic (workup/work up) was ordered.

Directions (6–10): Insert all missing punctuation in the following sentences, including commas, semicolons, hyphens, and apostrophes.

6. Mrs. Smith an elderly white female completed a marathon last week.

7. She ate two chocolate chip cookies however she did not feel any better.

8. The 1 cm paper cut was closed with figure of eight sutures.

9. He was therefore sent home to his mother.

10. He should be able to resume quilting in two weeks time.

Directions (11–15): Choose the correct answer from the choices given.

11. The hormone-producing cells of the pancreas are called _____.

    a. Meibomian glands

    b. Islets of Langerhans

    c. Corpus callosum

    d. Paneth cells

12. A very small bone is a(n) _____.

    a. Ossicle

    b. Tubercle

    c. Leuteum

    d. Curette

13. The process of belching is called _____.

    a. Borborygmus

    b. Eructation

    c. Flatulence

    d. Palsy

14. Repeating back the same words spoken to you is called _____.

    a. Verbigeration

    b. Misocainea

    c. Echolalia

    d. Xanthoma

15. Which of the following is/are used to diagnose medical conditions?

    a. Chandelier sign

    b. Froment paper sign

    c. Doll's eyes sign

    d. Mulder's clunk

    e. All of the above

Now, check your answers:

1. followup

2. mucous

3. affect

4. cord

5. workup

6. Mrs. Smith, an elderly white female, completed a marathon last week.

7. She ate two chocolate-chip cookies; however, she did not feel any better.

8. The 1 cm paper cut was closed with figure-of-eight sutures.

9. He was, therefore, sent home to his mother.

10. He should be able to resume quilting in two weeks' time.

11. B

12. A

13. B

14. C

15. E

Questions 1 through 10 check your English grammar and punctuation skills. As mundane as these topics may seem, they're essential for MTs. In only ten questions, it's hard to get a clear picture of your skill level, but here's a general guide:

✔ **If you got all ten questions correct,** congratulations! Your grammar and punctuation skills are above average. This will serve you well if you decide to become an MT.

✔ **If you got six to nine questions correct,** not too bad, but you'll need to do better. Fortunately, grammar, spelling, and punctuation are covered in detail in every quality MT curriculum, so you'll have lots of opportunity to strengthen these skills.

> ✔ **If you got five or fewer questions correct,** you have a lot of room for improvement. If you're willing to buckle down and do battle with comma placement, semicolons, and other minutiae of punctuation and grammar, you can probably overcome this shortcoming. If that prospect sends chills down your spine, MT probably isn't for you.

Questions 11 through 15 ask about medical terminology and trivia. If you missed most or all of them, don't panic — these questions are all about the process, not selecting the correct answers. If you got them all right, you either have an astounding reservoir of medical terminology knowledge or you used outside references. Even seasoned MTs can't answer all of questions 11 through 15 without resorting to references. If that makes you a little envious, that's a good sign.

With training, you can hone the medical vocabulary, grammar, and proofreading skills touched on in Part 1. Part 2 of the self-assessment explores less-trainable factors: your personality tendencies and lifestyle needs.

Part 2: Personally speaking

Directions (1–8): Answer yes or no to the following questions:

1. Did you enjoy Part 1 of the self-assessment?

2. Do you frequently notice small details, such as misspellings on business signs and whether the salt and pepper shakers on a restaurant table are neatly aligned?

3. Can you work under pressure and deal with deadlines?

4. Are you able to concentrate intensely for extended periods?

5. Are you comfortable working independently and with minimal social contact?

6. Are you computer savvy and comfortable with technology?

7. Do you have another source of income to rely on while you become a proficient MT?

8. Are you willing to invest the time necessary to undergo formal medical transcription training?

Your answers to Part 2 identify how well a medical transcription career would mesh with your personality and lifestyle needs. Here's what your answers reveal:

> ✔ **Did you enjoy Part 1 of the self-assessment?** Your answer to this question speaks volumes about your psychological suitability for medical transcription. If you've already planned to look up the medical signs in question 15, you have the curiosity and interest in medical science that

are prerequisites to a successful MT career. If, on the other hand, you were annoyed by being asked to define obscure medical terms and clean up sentence formatting, you're unlikely to be satisfied doing MT work over the long haul.

✔ **Do you frequently notice small details, such as misspellings on business signs and whether the salt and pepper shakers on a restaurant table are neatly aligned?** Although you don't have to be at the absolute top of the perfectionist scale, you'd better lean heavily in that direction. MTs must pay attention to every single syllable. Although specific techniques for keying in on erroneous details can be learned, to some extent it's an inherent personality trait that you either have or you don't.

✔ **Can you work under pressure and deal with deadlines?** Deadlines are a day-in, day-out presence in medical transcription — deadlines to transcribe a minimum number of lines in a specified period of time, report turnaround times that must be met, even emergency reports where a treatment (and patient) are literally waiting for you to get the report transcribed and back into their system.

Deadlines can be motivating — there's nothing like a looming deadline to cut procrastination off at the knees. However, whereas some people experience deadlines as a trigger to roll up their sleeves and get down to business, other people find just the opposite. When the pressure to produce quality work smacks straight up against an "or else" deadline, the resulting shock waves can be overwhelming and put a stranglehold on performance. You don't have to thrive under deadline pressure to be an MT, but you do need to be able to handle it without stressing out.

✔ **Are you able to concentrate intensely for extended periods?** *Extended periods* means hours at a time, eight hours a day or longer if you're working full time. If you're the kind of person who gets so wrapped up in a task that you lose track of time, this aspect of MT work will probably come naturally to you. If you can't go 30 minutes without visiting a social website or checking what's new on CNN, getting to your desk and staying there even on days when you don't feel like it may prove to be too great a challenge.

✔ **Are you comfortable working independently and with minimal social contact?** The home-based nature of most MT jobs today means that most of the time it's just going to be you and the computer. There won't be any co-workers to interrupt you with idle chitchat — but they won't be around to provide social interaction either. If you're a people person, you may find MT work unpleasantly isolating. A strong social network you can tap into in your off-hours will go a long way toward keeping potential loneliness at bay.

✔ **Are you computer savvy and comfortable with technology?** You don't have to be a technical wizard, but you will need strong basic computer skills. Fast keyboarding ranks near the top, but you'll also need to

- Learn new software and master its shortcuts

- Plug and unplug computer peripheral devices

- Be able to recognize and react to Internet connection issues

- Have a plan for when you need more advanced technical support.

✔ **Do you have another source of income to rely on while you become a proficient MT?** With very few exceptions, medical transcription isn't a career where you can start earning a living wage right away. As an entry-level MT, you can expect to be near the bottom of the pay scale. In an employer-employee relationship, you're guaranteed at least minimum wage from day one and can work your way up from there. If your first job is as an independent contractor, it's quite possible you'll actually start out earning less than minimum wage. You'll quickly pick up speed as you develop your ear for dictation and learn how to apply the speed techniques described in Chapter 5. If you don't have another source of income to draw on until then, though, you may find yourself in a financial pickle.

✔ **Are you willing to invest the time needed to undergo formal medical transcription training?** Despite what some magazine ads and seminars claim, you can't go from zero to working MT in six weeks by completing a course. At the bare minimum, plan on six to eight months, and that's if you're a very diligent student with plenty of time available to study. If you'll be fitting in your MT coursework around existing obligations, plan on one or two years.

Why Medical Transcription Can Be a Great Career

Medical transcription is demanding work, to be sure. It requires time, persistence, and intellectual and physical stamina to succeed. It's also one of the few careers you can craft to work around your life instead of the other way around.

You can train at home

Although completing a formal MT curriculum is not optional, whether you do it from home or in a classroom is totally up to you. It's not going to be a cake-walk either; extensive, diligent studying will be required, along with a significant chunk of change to pay for it. There are plenty of online MT schools and community college programs to choose from. They're not all equally good though, so be mindful and select one with care.

You can do it from almost anywhere

Most MTs in the United States work from home these days. You'll need a computer, foot pedal, Internet connection, education, and dedication. An MT job is quite mobile — take your computer and your foot pedal with you, and you can work from virtually anywhere you can get a high-speed Internet connection. If you need to relocate or you're with someone who does, you won't have to leave your job behind — it can come right along with you.

Working at home also means there's no commute time and no traffic other than the family pets between you and your desk. You can work in your pajamas or ratty sweatshirt if you want to.

To be a work-from-home transcriptionist, you'll need to devote substantial, uninterrupted blocks of time to your job. If you're picturing yourself working diligently at your desk while your young children play happily at your feet, it's not going to happen. If you're distracted or sleep deprived, you won't be able to tell if a mumbling doctor is prescribing Aquasol (vitamins) or Anusol (hemorrhoid cream) for his patient.

It's fascinating and intellectually challenging

If doing nothing but typing all day would bore you to tears, you should be smiling by now. Medical transcription challenges you to distinguish ilium from ileum and requires you to know that there's a pelvis in your kidney. It demands the ability to unravel puzzling dictation quickly. What you don't know, you must know how to figure out.

Transcribing medical reports also opens a brief window into other people's lives. It's sometimes sad and occasionally downright funny. That peek is both a privilege and a responsibility. Yes, there will be boring reports and even entire boring shifts, but most of the time your mind will be even busier than your fingertips.

You make a difference in patient care

Good medical records facilitate good healthcare. As an MT, you won't be the person deciding the best course of treatment for someone, but you will be responsible for accurately recording the details that may be relied on to make it. How well you do your job can positively or negatively impact the medical care an individual receives, so be sure to do it well.

Your work schedule is often flexible

An MT work schedule can be very flexible — just how flexible depends on the type of accounts you handle and whether you're working as an independent contractor (IC) or employee. Even in settings where a fixed work schedule is required, it doesn't have to adhere to traditional work hours. Emergency transcription is needed around the clock at acute-care facilities, and transcriptionists willing to work nights and weekends are always in demand. Non-urgent transcription is, well, not urgent. It doesn't have to be turned around as quickly, which means there's some flexibility about exactly when it's performed as long as it's completed within a set timeframe.

This doesn't mean that medical transcription is a "work whenever you want to, if you feel like it" proposition. You'll have to commit to a particular schedule or to performing a certain amount of work within a given time frame. The details, however, are frequently negotiable.

Nobody cares how old you are, what you look like, or how you dress

Burn the panty hose and donate the power-ties to the charity of your choice; you won't need them working from your remote office. Overweight or underweight, drop-dead gorgeous or ugly as a toadfish, as long as you do the job well, nobody cares. If your physical mobility is limited, it won't hold you back. Even individuals who are completely blind can become successful working as an MT by using adaptive equipment. The fact is, many MTs and their employers never meet face to face, so not only do they not care that you've got a tattoo on your forehead and only shower on alternate Thursdays, but they'll never know.

Chapter 3

Getting a Handle on Job Prospects and Employment Options

In This Chapter

▶ Finding where the jobs are

▶ Assessing the impact of new technologies and global outsourcing

▶ Evaluating your income potential

*I*s a career in medical transcription viable for you from a financial perspective? It may be a great fit for your lifestyle and personality, but the money aspect matters too, usually a lot. In this chapter, you get the scoop on where the jobs are and how compensation is determined. You also find the facts and figures behind the current demand for medical transcriptionists and how that's predicted to change in the future.

Where You Can Work

Every physician group, hospital, urgent-care center, diagnostic-imaging center, or other healthcare service provider is a potential medical transcriptionist (MT) employer. Each of these places generates anywhere from dozens to hundreds of medical documents daily. The blizzard of patient documentation never lets up. Somebody has to make sure that documentation is clear, error-free, and available to be pulled up on a screen or out of a file by the next provider in line. That somebody is usually an MT.

MT employers come in three basic flavors: physician practices, hospitals, and medical-transcription services. There are major differences among them that you should keep in mind when considering where you may work. Your choice of employer will define the scope of your job, including

✔ The quantity and types of reports you'll transcribe

✔ Where you work and what equipment you'll use

✔ Whether your work schedule will be flexible or fixed

✔ If you'll be expected to perform additional, non-transcription tasks and, if so, what those will be

For a physician or physician group

Working for individual physicians or a group practice is one of the less hectic ways to step into an MT career. You'll have a short list of report types to master — typically history and physical examinations, office/chart notes, consultation reports, and referral letters — and they'll center around a single specialty, such as internal medicine, orthopedics, obstetrics and gynecology, or oncology. The pool of dictators will be more manageable, and with fewer idiosyncrasies to deal with and not as many accents to learn, you'll be able to get up to speed faster. You may even get to know the physicians you're transcribing — a rarity that can benefit both sides and grow into a long-term relationship.

The less urgent nature of clinic transcription often translates to less pressure and more scheduling flexibility. If you work on-site (which is a very large *if* these days), you'll have access to other healthcare professionals who can help you if you get stuck on a tricky spot and a built-in supply of people to socialize with when you're not transcribing.

The limitations that make working for a physician or specialty group attractive are also, well, limiting! You may grow bored doing the same types of reports covering essentially the same subjects again and again. If you and your employer part ways, you'll be less marketable than an MT who has a broader range of knowledge and experience with more report types.

 If you opt for an on-site position, be sure to clarify upfront exactly what your duties will be. MTs who transcribe in physicians' offices or specialty clinics may do so as part of a larger job description that includes non-transcription tasks, such as office management or medical billing.

For hospitals

If you crave variety, appreciate drama, and you want to get lots of experience quickly, hospital or other acute-care transcription can be the ideal route to take. There's no toe dipping with this kind of work; it's a full-on, sink-or-swim plunge into medical transcription. You'll encounter the history and physical examinations, office/chart notes, consultation reports, and referral letters that you'd transcribe for a small practice, but instead of focusing on a single area, they span many specialties and subspecialties and are joined by a broad array of additional report types. The specifics will vary by facility, but among them will be complex operative reports; specialty procedures such as bronchoscopy, placement of nasogastric tubes and stents, and insertion of chemotherapy catheters; diagnostic results from EEGs, EKGs, X-rays, MRIs, sleep studies, and echocardiograms; birth and death summaries; and more. It's a challenging and intellectually stimulating transcription environment.

Acute care may be more interesting than clinic work, but it's also much more demanding. It comes with shorter turnaround times (TATs) than other transcription work, and MTs are routinely required to commit to working at least one weekend day. You'll encounter a great many dictators with heavy foreign accents and less-than-perfect English. To be a successful acute-care MT, you'll need to possess a broad command of medical terminology, reference often, and perform ably under deadline pressure. If you're up to the challenge, it can be the most rewarding form of MT work.

A lot of acute-care facilities outsource their transcription to a medical transcription service organization (MTSO). If you want to do acute-care work and you can't or don't want to find employment directly by a hospital, another route is to hire on with an MTSO.

Acute-care transcription has a lot to be said for it, but it can be like drinking from a fire hose. It's not for the pressure sensitive, and if you haven't had extensive MT training covering a variety of specialties, you'll quickly become overwhelmed.

For a medical-transcription service

Quite a few MTs launch their careers by working for MTSOs. MTSOs provide medical transcription services to healthcare facilities, allowing hospitals, physician groups, and other healthcare facilities to offload a function that was formerly performed and managed in-house. The MTSO provides the transcription platform and the people to operate it. MTSOs range in size from sole proprietors (this could be you someday) who service a few local clients to large businesses that serve hospitals and physicians across the United States and Canada. If you hear someone mention "the nationals," they're referring to the big ones.

MTSOs are a frequent jumping-off point because

- They have a lot of job openings.
- Virtually every MTSO transcriptionist works from home, a very popular place.
- You can find employment with an MTSO as a full-time employee (with benefits), part-time employee, or independent contractor (IC).
- You don't have to be physically located anywhere near the company headquarters.

Depending on the MTSO (and your agreement with them), you'll be assigned to work on one or more of their client accounts. Frequently, you'll have a main account (primary) you work on most of the time, and another account (secondary) for which you serve as an extra pair of hands on an as-needed basis. If your work queue runs dry, you often can jump to your secondary and find work ready and waiting. Your primary and secondary are not by any means set in stone; they may change from time to time, which requires you to learn new rules, new dictators, and even new report types, all of which puts a temporary damper on your productivity.

MTSOs that handle large accounts, such as major hospitals, tend to have a very large percentage of English as a second language (ESL) dictators, which many MTs find difficult to transcribe. Chapter 7 contains techniques to help with this.

Running your own transcription business

It's theoretically possible to graduate from MT training, hang out an OPEN FOR BUSINESS sign, and start your own MTSO. However, doing so is incredibly difficult to pull off, especially now that medical transcription has gone so high-tech.

Starting an MTSO from scratch isn't the only way to own and operate a transcription business; you could opt instead to purchase an existing MTSO and make it your own. If running your own transcription business is part of your big-picture plan, by all means, go for it!

The best thing you can do to bolster your chances of success is to learn how to be an MT first, preferably by working for someone else's transcription service business. Working for an MTSO, or series of MTSOs, will give you a feel for how MTSOs operate and give your MT skills time to develop. Even if you don't work for an MTSO, working as an MT in some capacity before branching out on your own is a good idea. When you have some transcription experience under your belt, you'll be much better equipped to pull together the technology, clients, and maybe even your own staff of MTs.

Your Job Prospects

Mention that you're considering becoming a medical transcriptionist, and within minutes — if not seconds — someone will inform you that it's an obsolete profession. They're trying to be helpful, but they're mistaken. Despite the advent of pretty-good voice recognition technology and electronic medical records, medical transcriptionists won't be inscribed alongside the Dodo bird on the register of extinct species any time soon.

Speech recognition technology (SRT) and electronic medical records (EMRs) are a continuation of the evolution that has been taking place since someone first carved a notch into the cave wall to record a birth. Their presence affects how medical transcription is performed, but they don't eliminate the need for it. *Remember:* To err is human; to really screw things up requires a computer.

Watching the occupational forecasts

Job growth forecasts are tricky things, but the U.S. Bureau of Labor Statistics (BLS) specializes in them. In its *Occupational Outlook Handbook,* 2012–2013 Edition, it predicts that employment for medical transcriptionists will grow 6 percent between 2010 and 2020. Although not a meteoric rise, it's headed in the right direction. The number of jobs for MTs is going up because the demand for healthcare services is increasing, and every office visit, test, and procedure will need to be transcribed.

Per BLS employment data from 2010 and 2011, the top five MT employers are

- Hospitals
- Physician offices
- Business services (this includes MTSOs)
- Outpatient-care centers
- Medical and diagnostic laboratories

Knowing the facts on speech recognition technology

The technological advance that's had the greatest impact on the medical transcription profession is the improvement in speech recognition. SRT systems feed verbal dictation through computer algorithms to generate draft text versions of dictated documents. The drafts are then forwarded to an MT, who proofreads the draft while listening to the original voice file and edits and corrects errors.

Speech recognition (SR), voice recognition (VR), automated speech recognition (ASR), and continuous speech recognition (CSR) technically have slightly different definitions, but the terms often are used interchangeably.

There are two types of SRT systems in use:

- ✔ **Front-end SRT systems** create a text transcription in real time as a report is dictated. The dictator can see it on the screen and has the opportunity to correct conversion errors as they occur and sign off on the report immediately. The SRT software adjusts and adapts its future interpretations based on the dictator's corrections, thus customizing to individual dictator speech patterns and becoming more accurate over time. Reports may or may not be routed through an MT for review.

- ✔ **Back-end SRT systems** work differently: Instead of creating the text draft at the point of dictation, the voice file is sent to a central server, which processes it and produces a text document. The conversion process is far from perfect, and every draft is virtually assured to contain errors that the MT must identify and correct.

Despite how error-prone back-end systems can be, they're by far the most widely used form of SRT in medicine because they're quicker and easier from the dictator's perspective. The process of interacting with a front-end system and supplying the real-time corrections it entails requires substantially more time than simply dictating a report.

The accuracy of the SRT conversion process, whether front-end or back-end, will never, ever be 100 percent. It can be substantially impaired by background noise, dictator accents, inability to distinguish similar-sounding drug names, and other factors — items a skilled MT can usually sort out but a computer cannot. Nor is a computer likely to notice if a distracted physician dictates information in the wrong section of a report or switches right with left somewhere along the way. Speech recognition simply can't produce error-free medical reports.

Going E: The move to electronic medical records

A second argument people present when they explain why medical transcription is an endangered profession is that the EMR is coming. EMR is not coming — it's already here. Whether they like it or not, under current legislation, hospitals and medical practices in the United States must start using EMR or face financial penalties. The penalties will be levied in the form of substantially reduced reimbursements for care to patients covered by Medicare and Medicaid, a prospect that has medical facilities across the United States ushering in EMR systems.

It's already apparent that adoption of EMR will have a substantial impact on the future role of medical transcriptionists. EMR replaces the paper forms used in medical practices with electronic forms that record medical details directly into a computer system, with no scanning or typing required. EMR comes with many benefits. Chief among them, it requires a lot less physical storage space, and patient information can be transmitted between providers without having to fetch, copy, and fax it first.

The terms *electronic medical record* (EMR) and *electronic health record* (EHR) often are used interchangeably, but they have distinct definitions. An electronic medical record is the electronic collection of information on an individual created and managed by a single organization — essentially, it's the electronic equivalent of a paper chart. An electronic health record is the aggregate of all EMRs for an individual, regardless of where each one originated.

Many healthcare providers are resistant to EMRs because they like the ease of data entry and low cost of their current paper systems. It's also a major expense to pay for the software, equipment, and training required to make the switch. Data security is also a concern, given how often computer systems are hacked.

EMR systems come in multiple varieties. Some EMR systems are strictly template driven and require all information to be entered using point-and-click forms. These are extremely constricting and make no allowance for physician narratives and analysis. Hybrid systems take a more integrated approach, employing templates and allowing voice entry of physician notes. Somebody with medical knowledge is needed to transcribe those notes, or at the very least edit the often shaky results of SRT. There are many dictators with such heavy accents or unrecognizable speech patterns that SRT will never be able to successfully transcribe their reports, whether they're entered via an EMR system or not.

The move to EMR is already impacting the role medical transcriptionists play in healthcare documentation, feeding a migration from typing in dictation to medical speech recognition editing (SRE). It's not making medical transcription obsolete, but it is placing ever-greater emphasis on the "knowledge worker" aspect of MT work over the verbatim transcription process.

Speech recognition and EMRs are having a substantial impact on the medical transcription profession. It's too early yet to tell exactly how it will play out, but the MT profession will evolve along with these technological changes, just as it has many times in the past.

Grasping the impact of global outsourcing

Everything else seems to be outsourced overseas these days, why not medical transcription? The same technologies that enable American MTs to work from home make it possible for MT work to be done anywhere there's a network connection available. The labor costs are lower, and due to time differences, work can go on while most American MTs are sound asleep.

Although healthcare facilities began experimenting with offshoring work to countries such as India, Pakistan, and the Philippines about 15 years ago, it's a trend that's reversed sharply. Companies that sent MT work overseas years ago have been bringing it back due to concerns about patient confidentiality and data security and problems with the quality of transcribed reports.

The tipping point came in 2010, when changes in federal laws related to protecting patient health information made compliance with the federal Health Insurance Portability and Accountability Act (HIPAA) an even higher priority for medical transcription companies and healthcare facilities. As a result, an increasing percentage of requests for proposals (RFPs) for medical transcription services specify that the services must be performed inside U.S. borders by domestic workers.

Your future MT work is not headed overseas. In fact, work that once flowed out of the United States is now flowing right back in again.

Financial Facts

It's interesting work, and there are jobs out there, but how much can you really earn doing medical transcription? The answer varies considerably depending on who you work for, what type of work it is, and numerous other factors. Plugging in all the elements that play into determining MT compensation may bring back memories of high-school algebra. Fortunately, MT compensation pay structures can be broken into pieces and simplified, just like those tricky algebra equations.

How much you can expect to earn

First the big picture: total compensation. The U.S. Bureau of Labor Statistics collects data from employers of all kinds, nationwide, and uses it to estimate pay rates for specific occupations. Because employers are the data source, these estimates don't factor in the earnings of self-employed workers, a category that many MTs belong to; however, it's still the largest pool of MT salary data available. Table 3-1 lists BLS mean and median wage estimates for medical transcriptionists as of May 2011.

Table 3-1	Estimates of Medical Transcriptionist Wages	
	Mean	*Median*
Hourly wage	$16.37	$16.10
Annual wage	$34,050	$33,480

Source: U.S. Bureau of Labor Statistics Occupational Employment Statistics, May 2011

In case your math terminology is a little rusty, average salary is calculated by adding up all the salaries and dividing the result by the number of people: (100 + 30 + 30 + 50 + 40) ÷ 5 = 50. Average salary provides a general idea of what someone in a particular occupation is likely to make. The median salary indicates the dividing line between the highest paid 50 percent and the lowest paid 50 percent. It's the salary that lands in the exact middle when you line up the salaries in numerical order. The median of {30, 30, 40, 50, 100} is 40.

Some types of MT employers tend to pay more than others. As a general rule, the more technical the transcription is, the more you'll be paid. For example, BLS figures show that MTs employed by general medical and surgical hospitals are compensated at a higher rate than MTs employed by physician offices. This is helpful to know because it can affect your choice of employers. Table 3-2 lists the top employers of medical transcriptionists, ranked from highest to lowest mean wage.

Table 3-2	Mean Compensation Rates Paid by Industries That Employ the Most Medical Transcriptionists	
Industry	*Hourly Mean Wage*	*Annual Mean Wage*
Medical and diagnostic laboratories	$18.16	$37,770
General medical and surgical hospitals	$17.19	$35.760
Offices of physicians	$16.35	$34,010
Business support services	$14.46	$30,080

Source: U.S. Bureau of Labor Statistics Occupational Employment Statistics, May 2011

The U.S. Bureau of Labor Statistics may be the largest collector of salary data, but it isn't the only one. Several websites publish MT pay information that's easily accessible online. One of them is Salary.com (www.salary. com), which publishes wage and salary charts generated by crunching data collected from employers. As of May 2012, Salary.com calculated a median annual base salary of $38,695 for MTs. Figure 3-1 shows the proportion of MTs at different pay levels. Salary.com charts are updated frequently, and you can view the latest figures at www1.salary.com/Medical-Records-Transcriptionist-Salary.html.

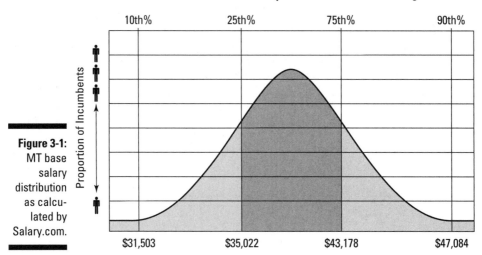

Figure 3-1:
MT base
salary
distribution
as calcu-
lated by
Salary.com.

Keep in mind that these salary statistics don't break out earnings by experience level. As a new MT, you can expect to land on the low end of salary estimates. Your productivity is likely to go up sharply as you gain experience, boosting you into the average or above-average range.

How you're paid: By the line or by the hour?

Now that you know the salary ranges for MT work, it's time to delve into the details. First of all, very few MTs are actually paid on a salary basis. Instead they're paid one of three ways:

- ✔ A set hourly wage
- ✔ On a production basis (how many lines you transcribe)
- ✔ An hourly wage with additional production incentives

A straight hourly wage is pretty rare. Most MTs are paid by the line, often with an incentive for producing more lines per hour. The line rate is called *cpl,* an acronym for "cents per line." For example, 8 cpl × 1,250 lines = $100.

Full-time medical transcription is commonly considered 1,000 to 1,500 lines in a day. Using the preceding example of 8 cents per line and 1,250 lines per day, the transcriptionist is paid $100 per day, or $500 per week.

A small change in line rate or your production speed can make a substantial difference in your income. Table 3-3 shows just how much.

Table 3-3   The Effect of Small Changes in cpl or Daily Line Count

	1,000 lines			1,100 lines		
cpl	Daily	Weekly	Annual (52 weeks)	Daily	Weekly	Annual (52 weeks)
6.5	$65	$325	$16,900	$71.50	$357.50	$18,590
7	$70	$350	$18,200	$77	$385	$20,020
7.5	$75	$375	$19,500	$82.50	$412.50	$21,450
8	$80	$400	$20,800	$88	$440	$22,880
10	$100	$500	$26,000	$110	$550	$28,600

It's important to note that the definition of what constitutes a line can vary from employer to employer. Employer A may consider 65 characters to equal a line, while Employer B says a line is 55 characters. Although that initially seems quite far apart, Employer A may be counting spaces as characters and Employer B excluding them, making the end results very similar.

A line rate that excludes spaces is sometimes referred to as *vbc rate,* or visible black character rate. A 55 vbc line is roughly equivalent to a 65 character line that includes spaces.

When comparing MT pay rates, it's also important to note that some employers credit the MT for all lines on a page, including page headers (such as report titles), subheadings, and footers. Other companies exclude everything but the report body from the calculation.

Be patient: It may take a few weeks or even a few months to get up to production speed. It's common for new MTs to start out producing 500 lines per day or fewer. A lot of your time will be devoted to getting familiar with the transcription platform you're working on and learning "account specifics" — special formatting requirements or transcription rules that pertain to the accounts you're assigned. At the same time, you'll face the traditional hurdles of new employment — meeting your supervisor, learning the processes for tracking your work and managing administrative matters, and generally learning the ropes at your new employer.

Quality and productivity factors

MT employers frequently add premiums to the base line rate to encourage speedy production. For example, a company may pay 7 cpl to transcriptionists who average 100 lines per hour but 8 cpl to those who produce 150 lines per hour. For every 300 lines transcribed, the faster MT would pocket $24, while the slower MT would earn only $21.

Quality is also a critical component of transcriptionist work. Reports are typically spot-checked by quality assurance editors, and the transcriptionist may receive a small additional premium, such as $0.0025 (yes, that's ¼ of a cent) per line for meeting quality goals, or perhaps a little more. Even though it's a tiny increment, if you average 1,250 lines per day, it will add $15.60 to your paycheck every week. Some companies go the other direction, docking the base rate for poor performance rather than rewarding high performance.

As in many professions, if you're willing to take unpopular shifts, like nights and weekends, you can expect to receive an incremental add-on for that as well. Chapter 15 includes pay-related questions you should ask potential employers to help you compare job offers.

Different rates for different things

Speech recognition editing work is frequently paid at a lower line rate than straight transcription, even if you're doing both types of work for the same employer. For example, you may earn 8 cpl for regular transcription but 5 cpl for SRE work.

Downtime is unhealthy for your paycheck

Linking pay to production definitely has positive aspects: If you perform better, you get paid more. If you want to earn more, you work more. If you have something you want to take time away from work to do, your employer (or client) is much more likely to accept that because they won't be paying you for that time, and you can make it up later (or ahead of time) if necessary.

The downside is that when you aren't producing, you won't be earning. As obvious as that sounds, it reaches farther than you might imagine. There will be times that you won't be able to work due to circumstances beyond your control. Your computer may crash, your Internet connection may go down, or your dog may need an emergency trip to the vet. Perhaps more frustrating, the company you work for may run out of reports for you to transcribe or its transcription system may go down, preventing you from working your usual hours. You may be required to make up that time outside your scheduled hours in order to meet your line count. You may be expected to sit at your computer and wait for work to arrive, without compensation for doing so. Any of these things can prevent you from transcribing and reduce your paycheck.

MTs often are compensated at a lower per-line rate for SRE work than for straight transcription, on the theory that it's quicker and easier to do. However, MT reports from the field consistently note that doing SRE work usually leads to a lower paycheck. For this reason, AHDI, the industry association for MTs, recommends that MTs evaluate SRE positions very carefully before signing a long-term contract.

Employee or independent contractor

An MT may be hired as an employee or as an independent contractor. An IC should expect to be paid a higher line rate than an employee would receive for the same work, because the IC takes on expenses that an employer would typically pay on behalf of an employee.

Being an IC essentially means you're running your own business, which gives you greater personal freedom but brings with it additional expenses and responsibilities. For example, as an IC, there is no employer paying payroll tax on your behalf, so you have to pay it yourself in the form of self-employment tax; also, whereas full-time employees may receive health insurance, ICs must buy their own. Chapter 19 goes into IC/employee differences in more detail, but essentially, hiring you as an IC instead of an employee saves the employer money and paperwork, and you should expect to receive a higher line rate in return.

Health insurance and other benefits

Paychecks aren't the only form in which financial compensation can arrive; benefits count, too. In fact, they can count a whole lot, depending on how good they are. An MT employer may be your ticket to obtaining affordable health insurance, disability insurance, even life insurance. If you've ever paid an entire health premium out of your own pocket, or gone without, you know just how valuable this can be.

Unless you're definitely planning to work as an independent contractor — in which case, you'll be responsible for providing your own benefits — they should definitely be factored in to any calculation of your MT earning potential.

Chapter 4

Becoming a Working Medical Transcriptionist

In This Chapter

▶ Breaking in to the field of medical transcription

▶ Finding out about training options

*I*n the United States, you aren't legally required to hold a professional license or certification of any kind in order to be a medical transcriptionist (MT). There are no board exams to pass or training programs or apprenticeships that you must complete. In fact, from a legal perspective, someone with absolutely no experience could tune up his résumé tonight and start applying for MT positions by morning. It would be an exercise in futility, though, because no one would hire him.

Although you won't have to scale a mountain of requirements to become a medical transcriptionist, you will have to leap a few hurdles. In this chapter, I fill you in on what those hurdles are and give you advice on how to propel yourself over them.

Getting off the Launch Pad: What You'll Need to Break In

Because you already meet the legal requirements to be an MT (that is, you're alive), you're in a perfect position to start tackling the real requirements. The first thing you need is formal training in medical transcription. No employer will give your résumé even the briefest look for the most entry-level MT job without it. The formal education bit isn't just there so you'll have something convincing to put on your job application; it's there because MT work requires you to know a lot of stuff.

As an MT, you're going to be elbow-deep in people's healthcare details — you'd better know what you're doing! In addition to covering the underlying knowledge required, any MT course worth taking will incorporate hands-on time transcribing reports from actual dictation. Practice is a key part of learning, and practice you will — a lot. Would you undertake repairing the brakes or transmission in someone's car if the closest you'd ever come to the innards of a vehicle was reading about them? Would you allow someone to work on your vehicle if that was their sole claim to competence?

What about on-the-job training? Can't you learn that way? To summarize: No. There was a time when it was possible — even desirable — to sign on with a healthcare facility, work on-site, and get trained and mentored until you were able to work independently. That's so rare nowadays that you can go ahead and cross it off your list of training options altogether. Healthcare facilities and transcription businesses don't have the time or resources to train lay-people in the intricacies of medical language, document formatting, and the other rules and procedures that MTs need to master. Employers expect MTs to be productive right away. Many of them are willing to hire trained but inexperienced MTs and nurse them up to full speed, but they won't train you from scratch.

The next thing on the agenda is a formal professional credential to go along-side your formal education. Although technically you aren't *required* to have a medical transcription certification, you may want to get one anyway. It's an option, and it's available.

The final items on your pre-launch checklist are patience, perseverance, and professionalism:

- ✔ Patience, because no matter what that glossy magazine ad or website promises, you can't go from zero to job-ready in six weeks.

- ✔ Perseverance, because you won't make it through all the coursework without it (though you'll be grateful for that coursework later). You'll also need to draw on your perseverance during the hunt for your first MT job. As with any career, finding an employer that's willing to take on a new graduate, and who you're also excited to work for, may happen quickly or require persistence.

- ✔ Professionalism, because office-casual applies to clothing style, not attitude and conduct. You may be able to work from home in your pajamas, but to get there and stay there you'll need to demonstrate discipline, integrity, and skill.

Educational credentials

To break into medical transcription, your résumé simply must include evidence that you've completed a formal medical transcription training program; otherwise, your application won't even be considered. Educational credentials are pretty much the only way past the tongue-twisting conundrum that applies to most professions: Employers want people with experience, but how do you gain experience if you can't get a job without first having experience?

A certificate from a reputable medical transcription vocational school or diploma from a community college medical transcription program are both acceptable options. Having one of these on your résumé doesn't guarantee an employer that you're competent, but it does provide substantial evidence in that direction.

Professional certification

As mentioned earlier, there are no licensing or certification mandates that you must meet in order to work as a medical transcriptionist. Nor is any potential employer likely to hold it against you if you don't have one, because certifications are far from commonplace among entry-level MTs. However, you may choose to earn a certification anyway, for a couple reasons:

- ✔ To potentially tip your résumé into the interview pile ahead of noncertified individuals competing for the same position
- ✔ To challenge yourself and see if you can pass the certification exam

Certifications vs. certificates: What's the difference?

Certifications and a certificates are entirely different things. A *certificate* is all about training. It provides documentation confirming that you completed specific training offered by the entity issuing the certificate. The training may be a full-blown MT training program, a single course, or even just a day-long seminar. It may or may not include tests. You'll receive a certificate when you complete your formal MT training and often for attending professional development activities in the future.

Professional *certification* is all about the test, which is carefully designed to challenge your MT skills. If you pass the test, you can call yourself certified. There may be ancillary requirements, such as pledging to adhere to a list of professional ethics. How you prepare for the exam, or if you prepare at all, is entirely up to you.

To ensure high quality, meaningful certifications, a rigorous process is used to pinpoint the material to be covered and create the exam questions. A statistical method called *psychometrics* is employed to evaluate the validity of individual test items and set a passing score for the exam. This is true of most professional certification exams, not just those related to medical transcription.

The only medical transcription certifications that are widely recognized and, therefore, worth considering are both issued by the Association for Healthcare Documentation Integrity (AHDI; `www.ahdionline.org`). They're currently entirely voluntary, though AHDI has been advocating to make them legally required. You don't have to be a member of AHDI to take the exams, but members receive significant price discounts. (As of July 2012, membership to AHDI costs between $55 and $135 annually, depending on whether you're a student, working, or not working as an MT.) The two certifications are

- ✔ **Registered Medical Transcriptionist (RMT):** This is the only certification that's realistic for new graduates of MT programs and fledgling MTs who have little or no work experience. The RMT exam tests core medical transcription knowledge skills expected of MTs who fall under the Level 1 category of AHDI's Model Medical Transcriptionist Job Description (see Chapter `www.ahdionline.org/ProfessionalPractices/White PapersResourceDocuments/ModelJobDescriptions/tabid/335/ Default.aspx`).

  The RMT exam consists of 130 questions covering three content domains:

  - • **Transcription standards and style:** These questions are about medical record types and formats, rules and standards for editing, grammar and punctuation, and similar topics.

  - • **Clinical medicine:** These questions assess your knowledge of terminology, anatomy, physiology, disease processes, laboratory tests, treatments, and other aspects of clinical medicine.

  - • **Health information technology:** These questions test basic knowledge of computer hardware and software, as well as abbreviations and definitions related to healthcare and transcription technologies.

  RMT certification must be renewed every three years, either by retaking the exam or by completing an RMT credentialing course that is offered only through AHDI.

- ✔ **Certified Medical Transcriptionist (CMT):** Newbies aren't outright banned from taking this exam, but it's intended for MTs with at least two years' experience in acute-care transcription or a multispecialty environment. The CMT exam steps it up a notch, testing skills that are expected of MTs who fall under experience Level 2 in AHDI's Model Medical Transcriptionist Job Description.

CMT candidates must already hold RMT certification. Optionally, you can take a combined exam, called the Credential Qualifying Exam (CQE) that covers RMT and CMT in one sitting.

The CMT exam consists of 120 questions that fall into two categories:

- **Clinical medicine:** These questions are about medical terminology, anatomy and physiology, disease processes, diagnostics, treatment, equipment and instruments.

- **Health information technology:** These questions asses your knowledge of terms and abbreviations related to computers, healthcare technology, electronic health records, speech recognition technology, standards, nomenclatures, and measurement systems.

CMT certifications are valid for three years and are renewed by earning 30 continuing education credits during the three-year cycle.

The following information applies to both the RMT and CMT exams:

- ✔ The exams consist of multiple-choice and fill-in-the-blank questions. For the fill-in-the-blank questions, test takers listen to a dictation excerpt, compare it against transcribed text that contains blanks, and fill in the missing items based on the voice file.

- ✔ Exams are administered through a third-party service. You can go to an authorized testing center and take the exam there or take it over the Internet. To take it via the Internet, you need a compatible computer and a webcam so the proctor can keep an eye on you as you take the test.

- ✔ The exams are pass/fail. Your performance on individual sections and exactly what the passing score is are not revealed. You'll get your results immediately upon completion of the exam.

- ✔ If you fail an exam, you must wait six months before you can take it again.

If you're considering earning the RMT certification, be sure to visit the AHDI website at www.ahdionline.org for the latest requirements, exam objectives, and costs, because certification programs, especially pricing, change from time to time. Table 4-1 details certification pricing as of May 2012. Note that candidates must apply for exam eligibility before registering for the exam. There's a $10 eligibility application fee.

Table 4-1   AHDI's RMT and CMT Certification Prices, July 2012

Credential	Members		Nonmembers	
	On-site Exam	Online Exam	On-site Exam	Online Exam
Registered Medical Transcriptionist (RMT)	$150	$100	$230	$180
Certified Medical Transcriptionist (CMT)	$200	$150	$280	$230

Avoiding medical transcriptionist "job" scams

Plenty of unscrupulous individuals prey on people seeking to do work from home, and potential medical transcriptionists are prime targets. There are two especially prevalent schemes to watch out for:

✔ **Medical transcription employment scams:** The scammer offers to give you on-the-job training; all you have to do is buy their transcription software and/or work for them for free until you become skilled, and then they'll start paying you. The only problem: Nobody ever gets good enough to get paid.

How they suck in victims: Through posting fake medical transcription "job openings" on job boards, luring unsuspecting victims to contact them.

✔ **Medical transcription training school scams:** Either the school doesn't exist at all, or it's of such poor or limited quality that any certificate you obtain from it will be worthless.

How they suck in victims: Through attractive websites, classified ads in print publications, or unsolicited emails offering to train you at home for a lucrative career in medical transcription.

Here are some things that should set your alarm bells ringing:

✔ **Training programs that promise to make you a certified medical transcriptionist:** No training program can deliver on that. The only way to become a Certified Medical Transcriptionist (CMT) is through the AHDI industry association, and CMT isn't available to newbies.

✔ **Inflated job outlook projections on websites offering to train you at home:** You may see a claim along the lines of "medical transcription employment is predicted to grow faster than average."

✔ **Training programs that guarantee employment on graduation:** No school can guarantee you a job.

✔ **Medical transcription job listings that include phrases like *training available* or *no experience required:*** Think about it. Why would someone hire you with no experience? As I mention earlier in this chapter, being trained by an employer on the job is a thing of the past when it comes to MT work.

✔ **Any "job" that you have to pay a fee to get, whether it's an application fee, a software charge, or something else:** No legitimate employer will require you to pay money to apply for a job.

In addition to being alert to these signs of treachery, stay safe by always doing your homework.

Don't rely strictly on testimonials or references provided by the company you're researching. Instead, check independent sources such as online MT community websites. Finally, trust your instincts — if something sounds fishy or too good to be true, it probably is.

Getting Educated

Building a solid base of medical knowledge and transcription skill is the most important thing you can do to break into the medical transcription field and stay there. You'll really, truly benefit from the training, and you absolutely need it to do the job. You'll study anatomy and physiology, medical terminology, formatting of the different report types, and many more skills you may not anticipate needing but definitely will need.

Legitimate medical transcription training programs are available through community colleges and distance-learning programs. Depending on your choice of program, you'll receive a diploma, a certificate, or a two-year associate's degree upon completion. If you're a very dedicated student, you may be able to complete a self-paced program in a shorter time, but expect to spend a bare minimum of nine months preparing for your new career, quite likely more. If you'll be squeezing studying in around another job or busy family life, plan for at least a year or longer.

If you already work in a medical office or have other medical experience, you may be able to take shortcuts and skip particular courses. Occasionally people somehow manage to move into medical transcription without formal education, but it's extremely rare.

Scoping out the medical transcriptionist curriculum

Although the details vary by program, any medical transcription program worth considering will include the following subjects:

✔ **English grammar and punctuation:** In particular, the program will focus on how grammar and punctuation relates to commonly dictated sentence and phrase structures and standards for transcribing them in medical documents.

✓ **Medical terminology:** You'll need to build an extensive medical vocabulary across a wide array of specialties, including medical prefixes, word roots, and suffixes and how they're combined. Coursework will also cover acronyms, eponyms, and Greek and Latin terms often used in medical documents.

✓ **Medical science:** The program will provide broad coverage of anatomy and physiology; laboratory tests and diagnostic procedures; pharmacology concepts and terminology, including drug forms and dosages; common diseases and disease processes; and surgical and medical procedures and equipment.

✓ **Formatting and styles for transcribing healthcare documents:** You'll learn about the structure and elements of the most frequently dictated reports and receive instruction on how to transcribe ratios, when to use Roman numerals instead of Arabic numbers, proper use of eponyms, and other details of adhering to healthcare document guidelines.

✓ **Referencing skills:** You'll learn how to make judicious and effective use of medical reference materials.

✓ **Computer and transcription technology:** You'll learn how to operate computer software and hardware and specialized transcription equipment, as well as keyboarding and word processing skills.

✓ **Legal and ethical issues related to healthcare documentation:** The program will cover HIPAA regulations covering patient privacy and confidentiality and how to deal with ethical quandaries you may encounter.

✓ **Practice, practice, and more practice:** Any program that doesn't include a substantial amount of time (hours and hours) transcribing actual medical dictation is not worth considering.

You won't necessarily take an individual class for each of the preceding areas, but all these subjects should be incorporated into the curriculum in some manner. As with certificate and degree programs for many fields, the specifics of a medical transcription training curriculum are crafted by the organization that offers it, making each one unique.

While there isn't an industry-wide, mandatory curriculum, there are two that you'll run across during your education research: the SUM Program and the AHDI Model Curriculum for Medical Transcription. A training program doesn't have to incorporate either of these curricula to be good, but many of them do so to some degree.

The SUM Program

The SUM Program is a medical transcription training curriculum created by Health Professions Institute (HPI). SUM is an acronym for Systems Unit

Method, and the core of the SUM Program is a package of actual physician dictations grouped into units by body system or medical specialty. MT students transcribe them to develop and practice transcription skills. The dictations come with answer keys so students or instructors can check their work. These dictations are essentially the de facto standard for transcription practice.

The SUM Program also includes a course syllabus, study assignments, and a matching list of textbooks that either are required in order to follow the syllabus or are recommended as additional resources. Many MT training programs incorporate part or all of the SUM Program into their transcription curriculum.

Why shouldn't you go straight to HPI for your MT training and bypass the middleman? HPI isn't a medical transcription training school and doesn't operate a medical transcription training school. Although you could purchase a copy of the SUM Program and follow it on your own, it's not a very realistic route to take. You'd have to purchase all the supporting textbooks and reference books separately and work through the very in-depth curriculum and often complex assignments with no support or mentorship. Even if you somehow managed to make it through the entire program under your own power, you'd be flying solo during the job search process, and you'd miss out on the connections many MT schools have within the industry. Those connections can be make-or-break resources when it comes time to land your first MT position.

AHDI Model Curriculum for Medical Transcription

The second training model you're likely encounter is the AHDI Model Curriculum for Medical Transcription developed by the AHDI industry association. Unlike the SUM Program, it isn't a physical product and doesn't contain assignments. In fact, it recommends the SUM Program for practice dictation. The AHDI Model Curriculum is simply a free, downloadable blueprint for training medical transcriptionists.

Seeing where you can study

There are two primary sources of medical transcription education: community colleges and online schools. Each has distinct characteristics.

Community colleges

If you're looking for a low-cost alternative that proceeds at a pace compatible with a full-time job or family commitments, a community college may be the best choice. Community colleges have long been the traditional first stop when training for a profession that doesn't require a four-year degree, and many of them offer medical transcription training programs. Although some community colleges offer MT training online, training in a traditional class-room setting is more common.

Community college programs may lead to an associate's degree, although many result in a certificate or diploma instead. Don't get too hung up on the distinctions between them — an associate's degree isn't any more valuable in the medical transcription job market than a diploma or certificate, and an associate's degree will come with extra course requirements not necessarily relevant to MT work. The main thing potential employers want to see is that you've gone through a reputable medical transcription training program.

The set schedule and predetermined pace of a community college can be constricting rather than ideal, depending on your personal preferences. Since community college programs typically follow an academic calendar schedule, there are usually only one or two times a year you can enroll. If a required course fills up before you can get in or isn't offered at the time you need it, your progress will hit a roadblock. The academic calendar can be your friend financially, though, because it means you have to commit to and pay for only one semester at a time. Increasingly, community colleges are offering MT training online, which can counteract some of the potential stumbling blocks.

Here are the benefits of community college programs:

- ✔ The tuition is affordable.
- ✔ There is a fixed schedule to help keep you on track.
- ✔ The programs are run by accredited institutions.
- ✔ They often include work experience opportunities through relationships with employers.
- ✔ You may be able to use federal financial aid programs to help fund your education.
- ✔ Because you register and pay for semesters one at a time, there is less financial risk if you cancel your MT plans.

And here are the drawbacks of community college programs:

- ✔ You can't proceed at your own pace.
- ✔ You can enroll only at certain times of year.
- ✔ You have to travel to the campus for most or all courses.
- ✔ There is a more complex and stringent admission process that often includes submitting a high school transcript, among other steps.

Online schools

Commercial training companies that offer online medical transcription home-study programs are more abundant than flowers in a florist shop. The most cursory online search will turn up hundreds of them. The ability to study anywhere (as long as you have an Internet connection), usually on a schedule of your own choosing, is very attractive, especially if you don't have a community college nearby.

There are quite a few high-quality, proven online medical transcription schools; there are also a lot of clunkers. Some of the clunkers are built by well-meaning but unqualified individuals, and others are just flat-out efforts to entice you to part with your money. Careful research can make the difference between graduating ready to launch your MT career or ending up very disappointed.

The flexible nature of online MT programs makes them ideal for people who are prepared to study hard but want to do it on their own schedule. You can enroll at any time, and the process is usually quick and hassle-free. Some online schools have a prescreening test to verify that you have reasonable English and grammar skills, but in many cases the only requirement is that you want to do it and can pay for the program. If you're a power studier, online programs can be quicker than the community college route. However, it's also easier to stall out along the way because you're responsible for setting your own study deadlines.

Home-study shouldn't mean alone-study. Any online course you consider should include easy, regular access to a qualified instructor and preferably an online student community you can participate in.

Here are the benefits of online medical transcription schools:

- ✔ You can study from anywhere you can access the Internet.
- ✔ You set your own study schedule.

And here are the drawbacks of online medical transcription schools:

- ✔ You must be totally self-motivated and self-disciplined.
- ✔ They're usually more expensive than community colleges.
- ✔ You need to exercise greater caution when selecting a school due to lack of accreditation.
- ✔ The tuition is less likely to be eligible for federal student aid programs.

Comparing your options

You may already have a strong feeling about whether you want to take training through an online medical transcription school or through a community college, but don't rush into either one without researching it thoroughly first. Be sure you can answer the following questions about any program you're considering:

- ✔ What are the details of the curriculum and where did it come from?
- ✔ How much practice transcription is included in the program?
- ✔ Have the instructors ever actually worked as medical transcriptionists?
- ✔ Are course materials, including textbooks, reference materials, and a foot pedal, included in the quoted cost? If not, how much will they add?
- ✔ How long does it take to finish the course? Is there a time limit or deadline specifying how long you have to complete the program?
- ✔ Is a computer with specific hardware and software specifications needed to complete the course? If yours doesn't make the grade, you may be able to simply upgrade it rather than buy a new one.
- ✔ What kind of student support does the school provide?
- ✔ Does the school provide any job search assistance to graduates, especially through relationships with MT employers?
- ✔ Is the school accredited? If so, by whom? (A no answer is not an automatic deal breaker.)
- ✔ What is the program's graduation rate? (This information is key. If a lot of students start the program but don't finish it, or if the school claims not to know the answer, be wary.)
- ✔ Can the program provide any statistics about employment rate for its graduates? (This information is very important, but it can be difficult for schools to track accurately.)
- ✔ What payment plans or financial aid options are available?
- ✔ What is the program's refund policy if you're unable to complete the program due to unexpected circumstances?
- ✔ When can you start?

Don't be shy about asking questions. You're about to commit a substantial amount of money and a great deal of your time. If you're too introverted to ask them yourself, get someone more outgoing to do it for you.

The "ships": Internships, externships, and apprenticeships

If you do your homework and compare programs from multiple schools, you may encounter programs that mention internships or externships. You may even come across references to medical transcription apprenticeships. What are these "ships" and should you sail on one of them?

The "ships" are variations of on-the-job training opportunities that allow students to gain practical experience in their new profession. Students work for free or below-market pay to gain experience working in the field. It's an arrangement that benefits both sides. The student, who is usually closely supervised, gets real-world practice, an opportunity to ask questions and observe, and valuable work experience to place on a résumé. The employer gets inexpensive labor and the opportunity to test-drive a potential future employee. It's not uncommon for the arrangement to evolve into regular employment after the student graduates.

The three variations you'll run across are

✔ **Internships:** In an internship, you spend time doing live medical transcription under close supervision, with minimal or no compensation and no guarantee of future employment.

✔ **Externships:** The term *externship* is frequently used interchangeably with *internship*. Sometimes it's used to indicate a shorter-term arrangement.

✔ **Apprenticeship:** A paid, extended variation of the internship intended to provide extensive on-the-job training. The apprentice and employer contract for a specified period, often multiple years, and a predetermined below-market pay rate.

In 2007, the now defunct Medical Technology Industry Association (MTIA) launched the only apprenticeship program for the medical transcription field. Few students were willing to commit to two years of MT work for minimal pay, and that particular ship sank.

Internships and externships are a bridge between the student and working world. They can be challenging to obtain because the employer has to devote a significant amount of time training and supervising the student. Although you shouldn't cross a program off your list for lack of an internship or externship, the inclusion of one is a definite plus.

Paying for your education

Before you tap out your bank account or even consider relying on a credit card (which is usually a bad idea), consider this: You may be eligible for financial aid.

The cost of medical transcription training can vary substantially between programs, but expect to pay $3,000 or more. Community college programs tend to be less expensive and are a pay-as-you-go proposition, allowing you to invest in your future career one semester at a time. Online medical transcription schools often require you to commit to tuition for the full program upfront, although they may allow you to pay it in installments. Either way, the costs can add up quickly, so it's well worth figuring out how you're going to pay the bills before you enroll.

If you attend a community college, there will be more options on the table than if you go to a for-profit medical transcription school. If you anticipate needing financial aid to pay your tuition, do your school shopping with that in mind.

Financing options can vary significantly from school to school. Ask schools you're considering what your options are — they should know what applies to them and may apply to you.

Expect the process of applying for financing — whether in the form of federal or state financial aid or a private loan — to take time. It's more challenging to obtain governmental assistance for career and vocational training than for traditional college degree programs, but it's sometimes possible. If you're in a hurry, paying for the training yourself will be the speediest and most hassle-free approach.

Hitting up Uncle Sam: Federal assistance

If you opt for a community college, you *may* be eligible for a Pell grant or federal student loan. Your school needs to be a participant in the program and you'll have to meet qualifications to be eligible.

Pell grants are based on financial need. They don't have to be repaid, and you must have a lot of need and very little income to receive one. Federal student loans are easier to get. They have advantages over most private loans offered by banks and credit unions, but they do have to be repaid. Federal student loans can be subsidized or unsubsidized:

- ✔ **Subsidized:** With subsidized loans, Uncle Sam picks up the interest while you're in school at least half-time; they're tied to financial need, but you don't have to be as needy as you do to get a Pell grant.

- ✔ **Unsubsidized:** Unsubsidized federal student loans also have favorable interest rates, but you're responsible for 100 percent of the interest. For unsubsidized loans, you're not required to demonstrate financial need.

With both types, repayment of the loan is deferred while you're in school at least half-time.

Federal and state financial aid rules and options can be complex and are subject to change. Be sure to visit the federal student aid website (http://studentaid.ed.gov) for the latest rules and programs.

To apply for federal financial aid, you'll need to submit a form called the Free Application for Federal Student Aid (FAFSA), which asks lots of questions about your income and financial situation. You don't need to pay anything or anybody in order to submit this form. Fill it out and get free help completing it at www.fafsa.ed.gov.

Tapping Governor So-and-So: State assistance

If you're currently unemployed and fit into the category "displaced worker," you may be able to tap funds available pursuant to the Workforce Investment Act (WIA). Displaced workers include individuals laid off from industries on the way out and homemakers who were dependent on a spouse for income but are now on their own, among others. The WIA program is administered though One-Stop Career Centers in individual states. Start your research at www.careeronestop.org or search the web using the name of your state along with the phrase "WIA one-stop."

If you have a disability, you may be able to obtain funding through employment services offered by your state's Department of Vocational Rehabilitation Services (DVRS). To find contact information, search the web using the name of your state along with the phrase "vocational rehabilitation."

Medical transcription education falls under the heading of career and vocational training, terminology to keep in mind while researching potential sources of financial aid.

Accessing benefits: Assistance for military members and their spouses

If you're a veteran, you may be able to use the GI Bill (www.gibill.va.gov) or other benefits from the Veterans Administration (www.vba.va.gov) to pay for your training.

If you're the spouse of an active member of the military, be sure to look into the Military Spouse Career Advancement Accounts (MyCAA) program. Details are available on the Military OneSource website (www.military onesource.mil) or by calling a Military OneSource Career and Education Consultant at 800-342-9647.

Taking out a personal loan

If you don't qualify for government-sponsored student aid and you're unable to pay for MT training from funds you have on hand, consider obtaining a private student loan from a local bank or credit union.

Take the time to read the fine print, even if you have to borrow someone's reading glasses to do it. Be sure you know exactly what the interest rate is, when you'll have to start making payments, and how much they'll be.

Part II
Getting the Job Done: Medical Transcription How-To

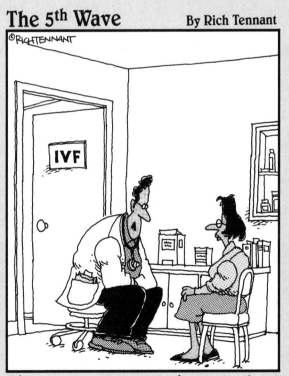

The 5th Wave   By Rich Tennant

"If you're going to transcribe for us, you should know that we endeavor to obviate perplexing verbiage to assist in making medical records less cumbersome."

In this part . . .

In this part, you work on five technical skills that lie at the heart of a successful medical transcription career. Chapter 5 provides a crash course in the underlying structure of medical terminology. Chapter 6 covers the mundane but essential topic of formatting medical documents according to current standards. In Chapter 7, you find out how to cope with the dreaded "difficult dictator." Chapters 8 and 9 get you up to speed on efficient and effective referencing and provide techniques to boost your productivity so you can work better and faster.

Chapter 5

Medical Language Boot Camp

· ·

In This Chapter

▶ Getting to know the language of medicine

▶ Identifying the parts of a medical word

▶ Building your medical vocabulary

▶ Avoiding word "gotchas" that catch less savvy transcriptionists

▶ Uncovering the Latin behind drug terminology

· ·

*U*nderstanding medical terminology will help you immensely in your medical transcription (MT) career. To the uninitiated, medical-speak may seem like an artificially complicated way to communicate, but actually it's just the opposite. By reducing potentially long phrases into a single word, medical terminology makes it possible to convey a lot of information efficiently. *Gastroscopy* is essentially a quick way to say "visual examination of the stomach."

The vast majority of medical words are simply combinations of reusable word parts. Both *gastroscopy* and *esophagogastroduodenoscopy* are built using the same pool of parts — one just uses more of them than the other. When you become familiar with the parts and how they fit together, you'll be able to construct and deconstruct just about any medical term you come across.

Just so you know, *esophagogastroduodenoscopy* means "visual examination of the esophagus, stomach, and duodenum." You'll rarely hear a physician actually spout a humongous term like that; they'll just use an acronym like EGD instead.

In this chapter, you see the basic parts that make up medical words and start building your medical vocabulary. You also get to know the abbreviations doctors throw in when dictating drugs and dosages. This boot camp isn't intended as a substitute for a full-length medical terminology course, but it does give you the know-how to recognize and deconstruct many medical terms and provide a solid foundation for learning new ones.

The Anatomy of a Medical Word

Nearly all medical terms are built using just three components:

- **Word root(s):** This is the main element of a term; it provides the term's central meaning. The root usually specifies a body part or system (for example, the appendix, urinary tract, blood, or skin).
- **Prefix:** A prefix can be added before a word root to modify the central meaning or make it more specific. It can add a location (above, around, inside), time (before, during, after), quantity (none, one, five), or status (new, crooked, fast).
- **Suffix:** The suffix adds further meaning, usually by specifying a condition (inflamed, painful, blocked) or something happening (removal, repair, examination).

Here's a real medical term, taken apart:

endocarditis = inflammation of the inner layer of the heart

endo- (prefix) = inside or within

card (word root) = heart

-itis (suffix) = inflammation

A bit of glue called a *combining vowel* often is added to make the parts flow together more smoothly. It's usually an *o* or an *i*. So, instead of, for example, *hepat* (liver) + *megaly* (enlarged) = "hepatmegaly," we have the correct term, *hepatomegaly.* A word root with combining vowel attached is called the *combining form.* So, *hepat* + *o* = *hepato,* and *hepato* is the combining form.

Take a look at how swapping out parts in this plug-and-play system alters the meaning of a term:

endocardium = the inner layer of the heart

endo- (prefix) = inside or within

card (word root) = heart

-itis (suffix) = inflammation

If you change the prefix to *peri-,* you get the following:

pericardium = the outer layer of the heart

If you change the suffix to *-itis,* you get the following:

> *pericarditis* = inflammation of the outer layer of the heart

If you change the word root to *hepat,* you get the following:

> *perihepatitis* = inflammation of the outer layer of the liver

The definition of a word part doesn't change, no matter what it's attached to. You can count on the prefix *peri-* to mean "around," whether it's *pericardial* (around the heart), *perinatal* (around the time of birth), or *perianal* (around the, well, you know). Similarly, the suffix *-itis* always means "inflammation."

To understand a medical term, slice it into pieces — prefix, word root, and suffix — and examine the parts.

Word roots: Brushing up on your Latin and Greek

You already know that word roots usually specify body parts, but why do they look and sound so . . . foreign? Who decided that the word root for "liver" should be *hepat* and the word root for "eye" should be *ocul?* As it turns out, ancient Greeks and Romans did. Most medical terms were devised at a time when anatomists spoke Greek or Latin. The word root for "liver," *hepat,* is derived from *hepatikos,* the Greek word for "liver." *Ocul,* a word root that means "eye," comes from the Latin word *oculus.* About 75 percent of modern medical terms are derived from Latin or Greek.

Table 5-1 tours common word roots by body part. Those handy combining vowels are there, too — tucked in right alongside roots that may need them. You'll notice that some organs have multiple word roots. For example, *nephr* and *ren* both mean "kidney." You need to know both because either one may be used.

The word roots, prefixes, and suffixes listed in this chapter are samplers of the most commonly used word parts. For the full menu, check out *Medical Terminology For Dummies,* by Beverly Henderson, CMT, and Jennifer Dorsey (Wiley).

Table 5-1	Common Word Roots by Body Part	
Body Part	*Medical Word Roots with Combining Vowels*	*Examples*
Abdomen	*Lapar/o, abdomin/o*	Laparotomy, abdominal
Anus	*An/o*	Anal
Aorta	*Aort/o*	Aortogram
Arm	*Brachi/o*	Brachioplex
Armpit	*Axill/o*	Axillary
Artery	*Arteri/o*	Arteriogram
Bladder	*Cyst/o, vesic/o*	Cystogram, vesicourethral
Blood	*Hemat/o*	Hematoma
Blood vessel	*Angi/o, vas/o, ven/o*	Angiography, vasculitis, venogram
Body	*Somat/o*	Somatic
Bone	*Oss/eo, oss/i, ost/e, oste/o*	Osseous, ossicle, osteal, osteomalacia
Bone marrow	*Myel/o*	Myeloma
Brain	*Encephal/o, cerebr/o*	Encephalitis, cerebral
Breast	*Mast/o, mamm/o*	Mastitis, mammogram
Cheek	*Bucc/o*	Buccal
Chest, rib cage	*Steth/o, thorac/o*	Stethoscope, thoractomy
Colon	*Col/o*	Colitis
Duodenum	*Duoden/o*	Duodenoscopy
Ear	*Ot/o*	Otic
Eardrum	*Tympan/o*	Tympanic
Esophagus	*Esophag/o*	Esophagitis
Eye	*Ophthalm/o, ocul/o*	Ophthalmoscope, ocular
Eyelid, eyelash	*Blephar/o, cili/o*	Blepharitis, ciliary
Face	*Faci/o*	Facial
Fallopian tubes	*Salping/o*	Salpingectomy
Finger, toe	*Dactyl/o*	Syndactyly

Body Part	Medical Word Roots with Combining Vowels	Examples
Foot	*Pod/o*	Podiatrist
Gallbladder	*Cholecyst/o*	Cholecystectomy
Gland	*Aden/o*	Adenoma
Gums	*Gingiv/o*	Gingivitis
Hand	*Cheir/o, chir/o*	Cheiroplasty, chiroplasty
Head	*Cephal/o, capit/o*	Cephalad, capitation
Heart	*Cardi/o*	Cardiac
Intestine	*Enter/o*	Enteroscopy
Jaw	*Gnath/o*	Gnathopathy
Joint	*Arthr/o*	Arthritis
Kidney	*Nephr/o, ren/o*	Nephritis, renal
Lip	*Cheil/o, chil/o, labi/o*	Cheiloplasty, chiloplasty, labiodental
Liver	*Hepat/o, hepatic/o*	Hepatomegaly, hepaticotomy
Lungs	*Pneum/a, pneum/o, pulmon/o*	Pneumatic, pneumonitis, pulmonary
Mind	*Psych/e, psych/o*	Psychedelic, psychosomatic
Mouth	*Stomat/o, or/o*	Stomatitis, oral
Muscle	*My/o*	Myositis
Nail (of a finger or toe)	*Onych/o*	Onchyomycosis
Neck	*Trachel/o, cervic/o*	Tracheloplasty, cervical
Nerve, nervous system	*Neur/o*	Neurology
Nose	*Rhin/o, nas/o*	Rhinoplasty, nasolabial
Ovary	*Oophor/o, ovari/o*	Oophorectomy, ovarian
Pelvis	*Pyel/o, pelv/i*	Pyelogram, pelvic
Pupil (of the eye)	*Cor/e, cor/o*	Cornea
Rectum, anus	*Proct/o*	Proctologist
Rib	*Pleur/o, cost/o*	Pleurisy, costochondritis
Shoulder, upper arm	*Humer/o*	Humeral

(continued)

Table 5-1 *(continued)*

Body Part	Medical Word Roots with Combining Vowels	Examples
Skin	Derm/a, derm/o, dermat/o, cutane/o	Dermatome, dermatologist, cutaneous
Skull	Crani/o	Craniotomy
Spinal cord	Myel/o	Myelogram
Spleen	Splen/o	Splenectomy
Stomach	Gastr/o	Gastroscopy
Throat (upper)	Pharyng/o	Pharyngitis
Throat (lower), larynx	Laryng/o	Laryngitis
Thyroid gland	Thyr/o	Thyroidectomy
Tooth	Odont/o, dent/i	Odontoid, dentist
Tongue	Gloss/o, lingu/a	Glossopharyngeal, sublingual
Tonsils	Tonsill/o	Tonsillitis
Trachea	Trache/o	Tracheotomy
Ureter	Ureter/o	Ureteral
Urethra	Urethr/o	Urethral
Urine, urinary system	Ur/o, urin/o	Urology, urinalysis
Uterus	Hyster/o, metr/o, uter/o	Hysterectomy, metrorrhagia, uterine
Vagina	Colp/o	Colporraphy
Wrist	Carp/o	Carpal

Prefixes: Looking at what comes first

A prefix modifies a word root's meaning. Think of a prefix as an exactifier, further identifying exactly which aspect of the body is being referred to. Prefixes can add

- Position (above, within)
- Direction (toward, through)

✔ Amount (some, all, one)

✔ Descriptive qualities (color, strength, size)

Prefixes are by no means required. Many medical words get along just fine without them.

Where is it?

Despite its small size, a prefix can dramatically influence the meaning of a word. The word *cardiac* refers to the heart as a whole, but *retrocardiac* means "behind the heart" and *intracardiac* means "inside the heart" — quite different places. Table 5-2 lists commonly used prefixes that specify position or direction.

Table 5-2	Common Prefixes of Position and Direction	
Locations	*Prefixes*	*Examples*
Above	*Super-, supra-*	Superficial, supraorbital
After, behind	*Dors-, post-, meta-*	Dorsocephalad, postnasal, metatarsal
Against, opposed to, opposite	*Anti-, contra-*	Antiseptic, contraception
Around, surrounding, near	*Circum-, peri-*	Circumcision, pericardium
Away from (separate, off)	*Ab-*	Abduction, abnormal
Away from, out of	*E-, ec-, ex-*	Everted, ectopic, external
Backward, behind	*Retro-*	Retroversion, retroperitoneal
Before, in front	*Ante-, pre-, pro-*	Antepartum, prenatal, procephalic
Beneath	*Infra-*	Infrapatellar, infraclaviciular
Beside	*Para-*	Paratracheal
Between	*Inter-*	Interarticular, intervertebral
In, into	*En-, in-*	Encephalopathy, incise
Middle	*Meso-*	Mesoderm, mesoenteric
Through, across	*Trans-*	Transfusion, transdermal
Through, throughout	*Per-*	Peroral, percutaneous
Through, during, across	*Dia-*	Diarrhea, diaphoresis

(continued)

Table 5-2 *(continued)*

Locations	Prefixes	Examples
Toward (near)	*Ad-*	Adduction, adrenal
Under	*Sub-*	Subgastric, subhepatic
Under, lower	*Cata-*	Catatonic, cataract
Upon, above	*Epi-*	Epidural, epicardium
Within	*Intra-*	Intrahepatic, intracellular

How much are we talking about?

A prefix can specify a quantity or amount. For example, *arthritis* means "inflammation of one or more joints," *monoarthritis* means "inflammation of only one joint," *polyarthritis* means "inflammation of multiple joints," and *panarthritis* means "inflammation of all joints or all layers of a joint."

Table 5-3 lists commonly used prefixes that specify quantity or amount.

Table 5-3   Common Prefixes of Quantity

Quantities	Prefixes	Examples
All, entire	*Pan-*	Pananxiety, panarthritis
Few, scanty	*Oligo-*	Oligomenorrhea, oliguria
Multiple, many	*Multi-, poly-*	Multiparous, polycystic
Above, excessive	*Hyper-*	Hypertherma, hyperacusis
Under, deficient	*Hypo-*	Hypotensive, hypothyroidism
Double	*Diplo-*	Diplopia
Equal	*Iso-*	Isotonic
Half, partly	*Semi-*	Semicomatose, semicircle
One	*Mono-, uni-*	Monocular, unilateral
Two	*Bi-*	Bilateral, bifurcated
Three	*Tri-*	Trileafleat, trigeminal
Four	*Quadri-, quadro-*	Quadriceps, quadruple

What is it like?

Prefixes can provide all kinds of descriptive details about appearance or state. For example, tachypnea means "abnormally rapid breathing," *bradypnea* means "abnormally slow breathing," and *apnea* means "no breathing."

Table 5-4 lists common descriptive prefixes.

Table 5-4	Common Descriptive Prefixes	
Descriptions	*Prefixes*	*Examples*
Absent, lack of, without	*A-, an-*	Apnea, anesthesia
Abnormal, difficult, painful	*Dys-*	Dyspnea, dyspepsia
Bad	*Mal-*	Malodor, malocclusion
Bent, crooked	*Kyph-*	Kyphoscoliosis
Cold	*Cryo-*	Cryogenic, cryoablation
Dead	*Necro-*	Necrotic, necropsy
Fast, rapid	*Tachy-*	Tachycardia, tachyarrythmia
Hard	*Sclero-*	Sclerosis, scleroderma
Large	*Macro-, mega-, megalo-*	Macrocephaly, megacolon, megalomania
New, recent	*Neo-*	Neonatal, neoplasm
Not	*Il-, im-, in-, ir-*	Illogical, immature, incompatible, irrational
Opposite, against	*Anti-*	Antibiotic, antiemetic
Separate, apart	*Dis-*	Disability, dissection
Short	*Brachy-*	Brachycephalic, brachytherapy
Slow	*Brady-*	Bradypnea, bradycardia
Small	*Micro-*	Microcephaly, microsomia
Straight	*Ortho-*	Orthodontist, orthopedic
Well, normal	*Eu-*	Euthymia, eukinesia

Something as basic as color can be used distinguish one body component from another. *Erythrocytes* (red blood cells) are distinct from *leukocytes* (white blood cells). Table 5-5 lists prefixes that specify color.

Table 5-5	Common Color Prefixes	
Definitions	*Prefix*	*Example*
Black or dark	*Melan-*	Melanin
Blue	*Cyan-*	Cyanotic
Gray	*Glauc-*	Glaucoma
Green	*Chlor-*	Chloroma
Red	*Erythr-*	Erythrocyte
White, colorless	*Leuc-, leuk-*	Leucomethylene, leukemia
Yellow	*Xanth-*	Xanthoma

Word endings: There's a suffix for that

Every medical word has a suffix. It's always the last part of a word, and its meaning never changes, no matter which word root it's attached to. A gracious plenty are just shorthand for "of or pertaining to":

-ac (cardiac)   -al (cervical)   -ar (ocular)

-ary (axillary)   -eal (esophageal)   -ial (myocardial)

-ic (pelvic)   -ine (intestine)   -ior (anterior)

-ous (cancerous)   -tic (antibiotic)

Telling your -ectomy from your -otomy

Suffixes can look quite similar yet mean very different things. Consider *-otomy*, *-ostomy*, and *-ectomy*. They're just a few letters apart in spelling but have dramatically different meanings:

- **-otomy:** A procedure that involves cutting but not removal. In a gastrotomy, the doctor cuts open the stomach, perhaps to examine the interior, but not remove it.

- **-ostomy:** A surgical opening. A surgeon performing a gastrostomy creates a hole in the wall of the stomach, usually to insert a tube that can be used for feeding the patient or drainage.

- **-ectomy:** Partial or total surgical removal. A patient who undergoes a gastrectomy will no longer have a stomach.

Table 5-6 summarizes surgical suffixes.

Table 5-6	Surgical Suffixes	
Suffix	**Meaning**	**Examples**
-centesis	Surgical puncture to remove fluid	Aminocentesis, paracentesis
-cision, -otomy, -section	Process of cutting	Incision, laparotomy, dissection
-desis	Fixation or binding of a bone or joint	Tenodesis, arthrodesis
-ectomy	Surgical removal of part or all	Appendectomy, tonsillectomy
-ostomy, -stomy	Artificial or surgical opening	Tracheostomy, colostomy
-rraphy	Suturing (repairing)	Herniorraphy, colporraphy
-pexy, -pexis	Surgical fixation	Nephropexy, splenopexis
-plasty	Surgical repair	Rhinoplasty, angioplasty

Suffixes you'll hear often

Whatever might happen to the human body, chances are, there's a suffix to describe it. Some things tend to happen a lot more often than others, especially the things described by the following three suffixes:

- ✔ **-itis:** Inflammation. Practically any part of the body can become inflamed, as you probably know firsthand.

- ✔ **-oma:** A tumor or mass. Of note, -oma doesn't automatically mean cancer. A lipoma, for example, is a benign glob of fatty tissue. A carcinoma, on the other hand, is a cancer.

- ✔ **-pathy:** A catch-all suffix meaning "disease or condition of." Most body parts that can -itis can also -pathy, from your joints (arthropathy) to your tongue (glossopathy).

There are almost as many "disease or condition" suffixes as there are "pertaining to" suffixes. In fact, they're so common, that they're included in Table 5-7, alongside other common medical suffixes.

Table 5-7	Common and Just Plain Interesting Suffixes	
Suffix	*Meaning*	*Examples*
-ation, -esis, -ia, -iasis, -ism, -ity, -osis, -pathy, -sis, -y	Disease or condition	Paralysis, rheumatism
-algia, -odynia	Pain	Gastrodynia
-derma	Skin condition	Scleroderma
-edema	Swelling	Lymphedema
-emia	Blood condition	Anemia
-esthesia	Sensation	Anesthesia
-kinesia, -kinesis	Movement	Akinesia, hyperkinesis
-logist	One who studies, a specialist	Cardiologist
-malacia	Softening	Osteomalacia
-megaly	Enlargement	Splenomegaly
-penia	Decrease or deficiency	Osteopenia
-phage, -phagia	Eating or devouring	Dysphagia
-ptosis	Sagging	Blepharoptosis
-rrhage, -rrhagia	Sudden and/or severe bleeding	Hemorrhage, menorrhagia
-rrhea	Flow or discharge	Rhinorrhea
-sclerosis	Hardening	Atherosclerosis
-trophic, -trophy	Growth or development	Hypertrophy

Getting to the meaning

Now that you know the building blocks that make medical words, it's time to break out your word scalpel and start dissecting. Before you start slicing and dicing, here's a quick anatomy review.

A medical word consists of:

- ✔ One or more word roots, which usually name a body part or system
- ✔ Possibly a prefix that adds additional meaning to the root, such as size, shape, color, direction, or amount
- ✔ Possibly a suffix that either means "pertaining to" or specifies a condition or procedure

Usually, but not always, the parts appear in prefix + root + suffix order.

Many people find it easiest to decode medical terms in reverse, starting with the suffix and working from there.

In the word *suprahepatic, -ic* is the suffix (meaning "pertaining to"), *supra-* is the prefix (meaning "above"), and *hepat* is the root (meaning "liver"). So, *suprahepatic* means "pertaining to above the liver."

It's perfectly legitimate to string multiple word roots together, as in *hepato-splenomegaly,* which means "enlarged liver and spleen."

Here's another:

oto/rhino/laryng/ology = the study of the ears, nose, and throat

Take a stab at this one:

tonsillar hypertrophy

tonsillar = of or pertaining to the tonsils

hyper = increased or excessive

trophy = growth or development

Put them together, and you have a case of enlarged tonsils. You may need a tonsillectomy. Hopefully, figuring that out didn't give you *cephalgia.*

Commonly Confused Medical Words

Many medical terms are pronounced identically or so similarly that it can be difficult to tell them apart. MTs fondly refer to them as "sound-alikes." Spellcheckers won't catch them because they aren't misspelled words — they're different words. The only way to ensure the correct choice is to know the definitions of both. With practice, you'll do it without thinking. Here's a starter list:

Abduct: Move away

Adduct: Move toward

Accept: To receive

Except: Other than

Aphagia: Can't swallow

Aphasia: Can't speak

Arteritis: Inflamed artery

Arthritis: Inflamed joint

Axillary: Pertaining to the armpit

Auxiliary: Extra helper

BMP: Basic metabolic panel (a group of blood tests)

BNP: Brain natriuretic peptide (a single blood test for acute heart failure)

C&S: Culture and sensitivity (a lab test)

CNS: Central nervous system

Callus: Hard skin

Callous: Hard hearted

Dysphagia: Difficulty swallowing

Dysphasia: Difficulty speaking

Elicit: To bring out or draw forth

Illicit: Illegal

Facies: Distinctive facial expressions associated with specific medical conditions

Feces: Poop

Fascial: Pertaining to a layer of fibrous tissue that holds various innards together

Facial: A treatment for the face

Hepatic: Pertaining to the liver

Herpetic: Pertaining to the herpes virus

Humerus: Arm bone

Humorous: Tickles your funny bone

Ilium: Uppermost bone of the pelvis

Ileum: Lowermost part of the small intestine

Intra: Within

Inter: Between or among

Mucous: A particular type of membrane

Mucus: Slippery secretion produced by a mucous membrane

Malleolus: Ankle bone

Malleus: Ear bone

Palpation: Examination by touch

Palpitation: Irregular heartbeat

Peroneum: Compartment of the lower leg

Perineum: Region between the legs

Peritoneum: Abdominal lining

Pleural: Lining of the lung

Plural: More than one

Principal: Primary or most important one

Principle: Rule or code of conduct

Prostate: A male gland

Prostrate: Lying on the ground

Scleroderma: A disease marked by hardening of the skin

Scleredema: A very rare disease also marked by hardening of the skin

Shotty: Scattered and bumpy like buckshot

Shoddy: Poorly made

Ureter: Carries urine from the kidneys to the bladder

Urethra: Carries urine from the bladder to the toilet

Beware of first impressions and literal interpretations. A medical term may mean something entirely different than it appears to mean at first glance. For example, *stomatitis* means "inflammation of the mouth" (stomat/o), not of the stomach. Even trickier, *cardiectomy* means "surgical removal of the upper end of the stomach," not removal of the heart! *Cardia* is the anatomical term for the part of the stomach that's attached to the esophagus.

Drugs and Dosages

Many of the reports you'll transcribe will mention medications, and there are a couple key things to know about them:

- ✔ Most drugs have at least three alternative names.
- ✔ Latin abbreviations frequently are used to express dosage details.

Generic versus brand name

Every drug has at least three names:

- ✔ Brand (proprietary) name
- ✔ Generic (nonproprietary) name
- ✔ Chemical name

The brand name Tylenol, generic name acetaminophen, and chemical name N-acetyl-p-aminophenol all refer to the same drug. Dictators almost always stick to brand and generic names, possibly because they don't know how to pronounce or spell N-acetyl-p-aminophenol any better than you do (and that's a relatively easy chemical name to spell). When transcribing drug names, brand names should always be capitalized, but generic names should not.

Chapter 6 covers the ins and outs of capitalization and other formatting matters.

Dosages: How much how often

Although they're often used interchangeably, the terms *dose* and *dosage* technically mean different things. *Dose* means "the quantity administered at one time" (for example, "atenolol 50 mg"). *Dosage* means "the regimen of the drug"; it's usually expressed as quantity per unit of time (for example, "atenolol 50 mg b.i.d.").

Dosages usually are expressed using Latin abbreviations. In the preceding example, the abbreviation *b.i.d.* indicates that the drug should be taken twice a day. Table 5-8 lists commonly used abbreviations and English translations.

Table 5-8	Drug Dosage Abbreviations	
Abbreviation	*Latin Phrase*	*English Translation*
a.c.	*Ante cibum*	Before meals
b.i.d.	*Bis in die*	Twice a day
h.	*Hora*	Hour
h.s.*	*Hora somni*	At bedtime
n.p.o.	*Nil per os*	Nothing by mouth
o.d.*	*Oculus dexter*	Right eye
o.s.*	*Oculus sinister*	Left eye
o.u.*	*Oculus uterque*	Both eyes
p.o.	*Per os*	By mouth
o.d.*	*omni die*	Every day or once daily
p.r.n.	*Pro re nata*	As needed
q.a.m.	*Quaque ante meridiem*	Every morning
q.p.m.	*Quaque die post meridiem*	Every evening
q.h.	*Quaque hora*	Every hour
q.4 h.	*Quaque 4 hora*	Every 4 hours
q.i.d.	*Quattuorr in die*	Four times a day
q.d.*	*Quaque die*	One a day
q.o.d.*	*Quaque altera die*	Every other day
t.i.d.	Ter in die	Three times a day

* Considered a dangerous abbreviation because it's prone to misinterpretation or has an ambiguous meaning. For the sake of patient safety, you should avoid using this abbreviation and stick to the English translation for the term instead. In rare cases, a transcription client may have a rule prohibiting you from making the switch, but that's pretty unusual. Chapter 6 goes into more detail on how to avoid dangerous abbreviations.

Getting dictated medications right isn't always easy. You'll have to pick out and recognize Latin abbreviations, multiple names, and numbers. Chapter 8 provides tips to help you nail down drugs and dosages and ensure you're transcribing them correctly.

Chapter 6

Formatting: The Basics

. . . .

. . . .

*I*f punctuation, capitalization, and spelling skills are not among your natural talents, you're not alone. Even high-ranking members of the Word Police can't remember all the rules all the time. Nonetheless, healthcare documents must be clear, unambiguous, and well organized. The dictator bears a responsibility to dictate reports in an accurate and comprehensible fashion, but let's face it: Your fingers on the keyboard is where the rubber really meets the road.

The issues of style and formatting are so important that there's a book over 500 pages long dedicated to it: *The Book of Style for Medical Transcription,* published the Association for Healthcare Documentation Integrity (AHDI). It's called the BOS for short. You and the BOS will most likely be spending a lot of time together.

The BOS is a reference book, and you'll only need to crack it open when you have to look something up. AHDI designed the BOS to make locating information as speedy and painless as possible; however, it's even quicker to not need to look things up in the first place. This chapter gives you the nutshell version of how to capitalize, punctuate, and format the things you'll encounter on a daily basis. Get a good grasp on these styles and standards, and you won't have to deal with the BOS as often.

Comma trauma: Why formatting matters

Improper use of punctuation or formatting can completely change the meaning of a sentence. Proper use, on the other hand, removes ambiguities and improves clarity. Punctuation is powerful. Just ask Nurse Nightingale:

> Turn the Stryker autopsy saw on, Nurse Nightingale.

Excise one teeny, tiny comma, and it becomes:

> Turn the Stryker autopsy saw on Nurse Nightingale.

Or this unfortunate patient:

> The patient came in complaining of chest pain. An hour after, he died.

A minor punctuation mishap can transform him from human to zombie:

> The patient came in complaining of chest pain an hour after he died.

It's not just about periods and commas, capitalization matters too: "I live in the white house" and "I live in the White House" have quite different meanings. Failing to recognize and capitalize brand names may get you or your employer into legal trouble, because neglecting to do so violates a company's trademark rights.

Proper punctuation and formatting are about much more than keeping yourself (and the dictators you're transcribing) from looking foolish to future generations; they're a vital part of accurate and professional healthcare records. In addition to their obvious importance to patient care, the reports you're creating are also legal documents. They could end up in a courtroom, perhaps to determine whether someone will receive compensation for an injury or is eligible for disability benefits, perhaps poor Nurse Nightingale herself!

Formatting and punctuation do three simple things:

- ✔ Group related items
- ✔ Separate unrelated items
- ✔ Clarify meaning

Report Headings and Subheadings

A well-organized report has all the expected things in the expected places, enabling a reader to quickly locate specific information. Headings and subheadings serve as landmarks and provide the structure for everything else.

Although there is no universal set of formatting standards that every report must adhere to (yet), the differences in how facilities format reports are usually small. For example, major headings are always in all capital letters, but facilities may differ as to whether the data that goes with that heading is typed on the same line or on a new line.

There is a trend toward standardizing the headings used in medical reports. In theory, eventually all facilities will use a predetermined set of headings for each report type, format them identically, and place them in a fixed order. It could happen. Although healthcare providers, particularly physicians, are very resistant to being stuffed into a one-size-fits-all box, electronic medical record (EMR)/electronic health record (EHR) systems may force them there anyway.

In the meantime, report formatting decisions are governed by two priorities:

- ✔ Client preference
- ✔ The guidelines in the BOS

Note: The examples in this section follow BOS guidelines and common variations.

A major section heading should be in all capitals and on a line by itself:

REVIEW OF SYSTEMS

Many facilities append a colon, although the BOS doesn't specify it.

REVIEW OF SYSTEMS:

Depending on the type of report and which major section it belongs to, a subsection title may be in all capital letters or it may have only the first letter of each word capitalized. In both cases it should be followed by a colon and then the associated data, like this:

ABDOMEN: Soft, nontender. No organomegaly or masses.

Abdomen: Soft, nontender. No organomegaly or masses.

You'll find out more about which subsection title format to use where in Part III, which goes into specific report types in detail.

Subheadings may be vertically stacked, like this:

LUNGS: Clear to auscultation and percussion.

HEART: Regular rate and rhythm.

ABDOMEN: Benign.

Or grouped into a paragraph, like this:

Lungs: Clear to auscultation and percussion. Heart: Regular rate and rhythm. Abdomen: Benign.

The grouping style is determined by report type and section, and, of course, client preference.

In the ALLERGIES section of any report, any allergies the patient has should be formatted in capital letters so they jump out at the reader, like this:

ALLERGIES: PENICILLIN.

When the patient has no allergies, only the heading is capitalized, like this:

ALLERGIES: No known drug allergies.

Items listed under the headings CHIEF COMPLAINT, DIAGNOSES (all variations, including IMPRESSION), and NAMES OF OPERATIONS AND PROCEDURES, should be listed one per line. If the dictator numbers them, you should, too, but there's no need to add numbers if no numbers are dictated.

IMPRESSION

1. Status post fall resulting in right digital radius fracture.

2. Multiple lacerations due to dog bite.

Acronyms aren't permitted in headings, so you should spell them out. Thus, a heading dictated as "HPI" would be transcribed:

HISTORY OF PRESENT ILLNESS

Different dictators may use alternative headings to refer to the same report sections. Where one dictator says "review of systems" another may say "review of symptoms." Transcribe it as dictated unless specifically instructed otherwise.

The heavy emphasis on formatting documents "just so" can stress out a new medical transcriptionist (MT) who is unsure whether to capitalize a particular subheading or append a colon. Fortunately, there's an easy solution: Look at previous reports from the same facility and format yours the same way.

Capitalization

Capitalizing a word boosts its visibility, raising it above the surrounding clutter of lowercase letters. The same rules of capitalization that applied in English class apply to medical transcription. This section focuses on how capitalization rules come into play in medical reports.

Drugs, diseases, and organisms

Capitalize the brand name of a drug but not the generic name:

> She is on Tylenol, Motrin, and Lopressor (brand names).

> She is on acetaminophen, ibuprofen, and metoprolol (generic names).

Don't capitalize nouns associated with the drug: Tylenol capsules.

See Chapter 5 for the meaning and proper formatting of abbreviations related to drug terminology.

Capitalize eponyms but not words that are derived from them. The language of medicine is chock-a-block with diseases, surgical procedures, tests, and equipment named after people who invented, created, discovered, or suffered from this or that. When the name of something is derived from or based on the name of a person, it's called an *eponym,* and it should be capitalized. Note that only the name is capitalized; the word that follows it is not. Here are some examples:

> Foley catheter

> Wolff-Parkinson-White syndrome

> Whipple procedure

Words derived from eponyms should not be capitalized:

Eponym	*Words derived from eponyms*
Gram stain	gram-negative bacteria
Parkinson disease	parkinsonism

Note also that eponyms are not written in a possessive format. So, the correct term is *Parkinson disease* not *Parkinson's disease.*

Capitalize the organism genus when the species is present. It's only a matter of time before you start encountering E coli, staphylococcus, and other organisms with Latin names. If both the *genus* (the first part of the name) and the *species* (the second part of the name) are present, always capitalize the genus but not the species, even if the genus is abbreviated:

> Streptococcus pyogenes, S pyogenes

> Escherichia coli, E coli

Otherwise, don't capitalize.

Some facilities follow the convention of adding a period after the genus when abbreviated, in which case you would transcribe *E. coli* instead of *E coli*.

A word expander, which you'll most certainly use, will handle a lot of these rules for you. Type in the shortcut you created (for example, *strpy*), and it will magically transform into *Streptococcus pyogenes*. Chapter 9 explains how word expanders work.

Titles of people, places, and trademarked things

Capitalize proper nouns. The name of a person, place, or thing should be capitalized if it is a proper noun. As you may recall from English class, a proper noun identifies a specific (usually one-of-a-kind) person, place, or thing. The names and titles of people, publications, companies and institutions, languages, countries, races, religions, holidays, countries, cities, and towns are all proper nouns. Here are some examples of common nouns and proper nouns:

Common Nouns	*Proper Nouns*
doctor	Dr. House
hospital	Massachusetts General Hospital
periodical	*The New England Journal of Medicine*
race	Hispanic
day	Wednesday
month	March
holiday	Memorial Day
religion	Methodist

The names of seasons — spring, summer, winter, and fall — should not be capitalized.

Capitalize the names of medical departments but not the names of medical specialties. This one can be a little tricky, because certain words can be used to identify either the general name of a specialty (surgery) or the title of the entity that performs it (Department of Surgery). To add to the confusion, the title may be shortened to just "Surgery." There are a couple tricks you can apply when in doubt:

> ✔ **If the word can be replaced with a person's name and still make sense, it's referring to a department or division and should be capitalized.** For example:

- "She will be seen by Physical Therapy." If you substitute "Dr. Smith" in place of " Physical Therapy," the sentence still makes sense. Therefore, it is correct to capitalize it.

- "She was referred for physical therapy." If you substitute "Dr. Smith" for "physical therapy," the sentence becomes malformed. Therefore, "physical therapy" should not be capitalized.

✔ **If the word has *to* immediately before it, it's being used to refer to the entity and thus should be capitalized; if it is has *for* before it, then it's referring to the specialty and shouldn't be capitalized.** For example:

- The specimen will be sent to Pathology.

- The specimen will be sent for pathology.

Capitalize brand or trade names of medical items. Many medical items are marketed under brand/trade names, particularly medical and surgical equipment. When a brand name is used, it should be capitalized. The brand name may consist of more than one word; if so, all the words should be capitalized:

Medtronic Bio-Pump	Medtronic pump
#3-0 Vicryl sutures	#3-0 polyethylene sutures

It isn't always obvious whether a word represents a brand name. When in doubt, consult a medical word book or other reference resource.

Punctuation

Dictators dictate reports; MTs punctate them. Omitting a comma, semicolon, or other bit of punctuation may have little impact on a sentence's clarity, or it may dramatically alter the meaning. Consider the case of Dr. Jekyll, who appears to be a pretty helpful guy:

Dr. Jekyll sutures punctures and wounds.

Insert a pair of commas, and he goes from helpful to heinous:

Dr. Jekyll sutures, punctures, and wounds.

Few punctuation mistakes have such far-reaching consequences, but they all have the potential to wreak havoc on the intended meaning of a sentence. If you don't have a solid grasp on proper punctuation, a patient may pay the price for your error. Master the key rules in this section, and minimize chance that you'll be the one responsible for transforming Dr. Jekyll from good to evil.

Separators: Commas, semicolons, and colons

The most prevalent, most helpful, and most problematic splat of ink ever invented is probably the comma. Colons and semicolons are not far behind. Writers (and transcribers) tend to add too many rather than too few. The first step toward using these common punctuators correctly is to keep in mind that they're separators, not pauses. They're not intended to indicate a point where a reader should stop and take a breath (or where the dictator actually did).

Commas

Insert a comma before a conjunction *(and, but, or, nor, for, so)* that separates two independent clauses:

> She tolerated the procedure well, and she was taken to the PACU.

In this example, the clauses on either side of the *and* could stand alone as separate sentences; thus, the comma should be used. If one or the other could not stand alone, leave the comma out:

> She tolerated the procedure well and was taken to the PACU.

Because "was taken to the PACU" cannot stand alone, no comma is used.

Use commas to set off nonessential information in a sentence:

> The patient, *who is learning to transcribe,* has a colon problem.

> The patient *who is learning to transcribe* has a colon problem.

In the first sentence, "who is learning to transcribe" is a bit of extra information about the patient. It could be removed without changing the meaning of the sentence, which is that the patient has a colon problem.

In the second sentence "who is learning to transcribe" is essential information because it identifies which patient has the colon problem — the one who is learning to transcribe. It should not be set off by commas.

It's up to you to use context to determine which is intended and punctuate accordingly.

Use a comma to set off an introductory phrase or clause:

> After eating deep-fried Oreos at the fair, the patent felt nauseous.

Introductory elements often begin with words such as *after, about, although, because, during, since, unless, until, whenever,* and *while,* among others.

Use a comma to separate two or more adjectives modifying the same noun:

> This tall, anxious male came to the ER this morning.

> This is a well-developed, well-nourished female in no distress.

Exception: Dictators often use a string of adjectives descriptors to identify the age, race, and gender of a patient, and it is common practice in medical documents to omit the commas in this type of sentence:

> This is a 24-year-old Hispanic female with a history of migraines.

> The patient is a 66-year-old Caucasian male who appears very fit.

Use a comma to separate two or more items in a series unless they are all connected by *and* or *or:*

> He is complaining of nausea, vomiting, and fatigue.

> I advised her to take two Tylenol, elevate her ankle, and call me in the morning.

Don't insert commas if all the items in the series are connected by *and* or *or:*

> He is complaining of nausea and vomiting and fatigue.

There are more rules governing the placement of commas than any other element of punctuation. If you need additional guidance, hit up the BOS.

Semicolons and colons

A semicolon is stronger than a comma but weaker than a period. Semicolons are especially useful for separating groups of lab results and setting off that perennial favorite physician transitional word: *however.*

Insert semicolons between series of phrases or clauses when any item within the series has commas:

> Heart: Regular rate and rhythm; no murmur, gallop, or rub; normal S1.

Use a semicolon to separate two independent clauses connected by a transitional word or phrase, such as *however:*

> The patient was told to use crutches for 3 days; however, he did not.

If the transitional word or phrase appears in the middle of an independent clause instead of between two of them, don't use a semicolon; use commas to set it off instead:

> The patient, however, did not use his crutches as instructed.

There are many transitional words and phrases in the English language. The ones you'll encounter regularly include *however, therefore, in addition, otherwise, although, instead,* and *nevertheless.*

Use a colon to introduce a list. If a complete sentence ends with the words *as follows* or *the following,* that's a clue to insert a colon:

> His history includes the following: dyspnea, fatigue, and cough.

> His history includes dyspnea, fatigue, and cough.

Connectors: Hyphens and apostrophes

Hyphenate compound adjectives when they precede a noun but not when they follow it:

> The patient is a well-developed, well-nourished male.

> The patient is well developed and well nourished.

Don't hyphenate a word that ends in -*ly* with another word:

> moderately severe pain

Hyphenate numbers compounded with words:

> This is a 3-week-old infant.

> The infant is 3 weeks old.

Hyphenate the prefixes *ex-, self-,* and *vice-* and any prefix that causes an odd combination of letters:

> He is ex-military.

> We re-covered the wound.

> An anti-emetic was given.

Don't use a hyphen with common prefixes like pre- or post- when part of an adjective before a noun or when used in "status post":

> preoperative
>
> postoperative
>
> supraspinatus
>
> status post appendectomy

Per the BOS, the list of common prefixes includes *ante-, anti-, bi-, co-, contra-, counter-, de-, extra-, infra-, intra-, micro-, mid-, non-, over-, peri-, pre-, post-, pro-, pseudo-, re-, semi-, sub-, super-, supra-, trans-, tri-, ultra-, un-,* and *under-.*

This rule doesn't apply if the noun is capitalized (a proper noun or eponym):

> non-Hodgkin lymphoma
>
> anti-American

Use hyphens when needed to avoid confusion:

> A small-bowel obstruction (obstruction of the small bowel)
>
> A small bowel obstruction (a small obstruction of the bowel)

Use a suspensive hyphen when multiple hyphenated words in a row have the same base:

> Her scalp is peppered with large- and small-sized cysts.

In medical transcription, "follow-up" has gone hyphen-free, so you'll always use *follow up* or *followup* instead. Many MTs have trouble knowing which to use when. When it's used as a verb, it's written as two words: *follow up.* In every other instance it's written as *followup.*

Don't use apostrophes in contractions, spell them out instead. It is common practice to avoid the use of contractions in medical documents, so you should expand any you encounter: *I will* instead of *I'll, he will* instead of *he'll, it is* instead of *it's,* and so on.

Use an apostrophe to show possession:

> The patients (more than one patient)
>
> The patient's nose (the nose of one patient)
>
> The patients' noses (the noses of more than one patient)

Apostrophes also are used to show possessive forms of time:

return in 2 weeks' time *not* return in 2 weeks time

Use an apostrophe to pluralize lowercase and single-letter abbreviations; otherwise, don't use an apostrophe:

wbc's

rbc's

X's

O's

EKGs

PVCs

 Get it right! When to use *its* (which shows possession) versus *it's* (the contraction of *it is*) is a common point of confusion. Here's a tip to help you remember: *It is* is the one with the apostrophe. Since contractions are spelled out in medical documents, you should always replace *it's* with *it is*.

Numbers

Perhaps the greatest potential for documentation-related catastrophic errors lies in a misinterpreted or erroneous number. It's vital to transcribe them in the clearest manner possible. The following guidelines will help you do so.

Arabic, ordinal, and Roman

Most numbers in medical documents are written using Arabic numbers. Roman numerals are reserved for very specific cases. Ordinal numbers identify position in a series.

Arabic	*Roman*	*Ordinal*
0, 1, 2, 3, 4, 5, 6, 7, 8, 9, and so on	I, II, III, IV, V, VI, VII, VIII, IX, X, and so on	1st, 2nd, 3rd, 4th, 5th, 6th, 7th, 8th, 9th, 10th, and so on
zero, one, two, and so on		

The most common uses for Roman numerals are in psychiatric diagnoses, cancer stages, cranial nerves, EKG leads, classification of some types of fractures, and in specifying Billroth anastomosis procedures. When in doubt, check the BOS or another reference.

Guidelines for transcribing numbers

Leave a space between numerals and units of measure unless they form a compound modifier:

> It is 5 cm wide
>
> 5 feet 2 inches
>
> a 5-pound weight loss

Add a 0 in front of decimal point for clarity (0.5 mg).

When zero stands alone, unaccompanied by a unit of measure, spell it out:

> He has zero chance of relapse.

Don't begin a sentence with a number. If it's dictated that way, recast it or spell out the number:

> 10 mg of Adderall was prescribed = Adderall 10 mg was prescribed
>
> 20-year-old female patient = A 20-year-old female patient
>
> 12 of my patients are male = Twelve of my patients are male

Hyphenate numbers that are part of a compound modifier, except when the unit of measure is metric:

> A 1-inch strip of gauze
>
> A 3 cm laceration
>
> A 2 x 3 mm lesion
>
> A 27-year-old Caucasian male

Abbreviate metric units of measure and spell out nonmetric units

> 1 mL
>
> 1 cm
>
> 1 inch
>
> 1 pound

Spell out nonmetric units if no specific numeral is dictated:

> Redness extends several centimeters bilaterally.

Omit commas in numbers with less than five digits:

1200 but 12,000

Fractions

Use decimals to express fractions associated with metric measurements:

1.5 cm

10.2 g

Use mixed fractions to for nonmetric units of measurement:

1½-inch strip of gauze

the infant weighs 8¼ pounds

Spell out nonmetric fractions when they don't appear with a whole number or are not used as part of a compound modifier:

He smokes one half pack of cigarettes per day.

He smokes 1½ packs of cigarettes per day.

Hyphenate spelled-out fractions when they're used as adjectives:

one-half normal saline

the dosage was cut by one half

Always use decimal fractions with percentages:

one half percent = 0.5%

Pluralizing numbers

Use an apostrophe to pluralize single-digit numbers but not multi-digit numbers:

4 x 4's

a male in his 50s

a set of 6's

the 1970s

Ranges and ratios

A hyphen may be substituted for *to* in phrases but not for *through*:

> Every 2–3 days
>
> Every 2 to 3 days
>
> Monday through Friday

Use a forward slash when the dictator says *per* or *over*:

> A grade two over six systolic murmur = A grade 2/6 systolic murmur
>
> Fifty nanograms per milliliter = 50 ng/mL

Use a colon in place of the word *to* in a ratio:

> A 1:100 solution

Appendix B includes more examples showing how to transcribe commonly dictated phrases that include numbers.

Abbreviations and Acronyms

Many acronyms have multiple possible expansions. For example, PVD can mean pulmonary vascular disease, peripheral vascular disease, or premature ventricular depolarization. MTs expand acronyms, abbreviations, and other verbal shortcuts to eliminate misinterpretation of their meaning.

Don't expand an acronym unless you're certain of exactly what it means based on surrounding context and/or references. Never guess.

When to spell them out

The first time it is referenced in a document, an acronym should be spelled out. Thereafter, it can be referred to by the acronym without expansion

> The patient has dyspnea on exertion (DOE). The first DOE symptoms. . . .

Expand acronyms dictated in admission, discharge, preoperative, or postoperative diagnosis; consultative conclusion or impression; and list of operations or procedures performed, even if you've expanded them earlier in the document.

Dictated: Operation preformed: D&C

Transcribe as: Operation performed: Dilation and curettage

When to leave them be

Don't expand an acronym if it refers to a disease entity or lab test, or if it's more readily recognized by its acronym or usually seen as an abbreviation, such as AIDS, BUN, CAT scan, and MRI.

If an acronym is included in a facility list of acceptable abbreviations, it shouldn't be expanded, even if it otherwise would be.

How to avoid dangerous abbreviations

Certain abbreviations, especially those related to medication orders, can result in catastrophic, even fatal, consequences when misread. For example, IU (international units), which is a dosage quantity measurement, can be mistaken for IV (intravenous), a dosage administration method. Consequently, there are several formal lists of abbreviations that should never be used in healthcare documentation.

The best known is the Official "Do Not Use" List (`www.jointcommission.org/facts_about_the_official_/`) published by the Joint Commission (formerly the Joint Commission on Accreditation of Healthcare Organizations (JCAHO).

The Institute for Safe Medication Practices (ISMP) publishes a list that incorporates and expands on The Joint Commission list. Many items on the ISMP list are specific to writing prescriptions and are unlikely to be encountered when transcribing, but MTs should still be familiar with them. The current ISMP list can be found at on the ISMP website at `www.ismp.org`.

Use the preceding lists as a starting point, but be aware that individual facilities may have their own "do not use" lists and requirements that differ.

Chapter 7

Cracking the Code: Deciphering Difficult Dictation

In This Chapter

▶ Balancing perfection and productivity

▶ Conquering unclear dictation

▶ Understanding dictators with heavy accents

*O*ne of the most challenging and rewarding aspects of transcribing medical reports is taking a sentence that is barely distinguishable as English and determining exactly what the dictator said. Initially unintelligible and downright bizarre dictation will occur more often than you can possibly imagine. After you get past either chuckling or unleashing a string of expletives, the hunt is on to figure out what the dictator really said, and you're the detective. Because accurate records are absolutely critical to good patient care, you can't guess; you have to *know*.

It's to your benefit and the patient's to do everything possible to accurately decipher every syllable a dictator utters. In this chapter, you'll learn key strategies for understanding speech that is essentially incomprehensible to non-MTs. With these techniques in your hip pocket, you'll be able to eradicate all but the most intractable blanks from your reports.

Aiming for Efficiency

The battle to avoid blank spots in your transcriptions is well worth fighting, but you must wage it with productivity in mind. Doing the investigation necessary to decode one tricky dictation consumes time that you could be using to produce additional reports instead. Successful medical transcriptionists (MTs) know how to strike a balance between completeness and quantity.

Figuring out this stuff is often like solving a puzzle, and slipping that last piece in place that suddenly makes the picture complete is very personally rewarding. It gets even better when you become the go-to person to solve the puzzles others have given up on. Becoming an expert at filling in the blanks also will boost you up the MT seniority chain and make you more valuable in the MT marketplace.

This detective work has a downside, though: It takes time. In the work life of most MTs, time literally equals money. Because MT pay these days is usually closely tied to the number of characters and lines transcribed, anytime you're not pounding out the lines, you're probably not earning money.

Thus, when a dictator lists a patient's lab results while swallowing the last mouthful of a sticky bun, you may be tempted to leave a blank or flag that spot in the report for further review. Although this approach may seem like the easy way out, it's not.

Too many or inappropriate blanks will tarnish the quality score assigned to your work. If that quality score comes down, so will your income. On top of that, someone else will have to be pulled from her duties to try to fill in the blanks you left behind. When that someone listens to the problem section and deciphers it in seconds, it's going to be a major blow to your pride and probably annoy the diverted person and your employer as well. So, you must do your best to fill in the blanks without slowing your work pace to a crawl.

To excel at this balancing act of speed and accuracy, there are three main things you need to know how to do:

- Find accurate information
- Transcribe correctly
- Work quickly

Fortunately for modern MTs, we have many more transcription tools at our disposal than our predecessors did. You may not be able to turn to a master MT sitting next to you who has been transcribing the very same doctor for two years and ask, "What did he just say?" but you have the entire web at your fingertips, dozens of reference books created with the sole purpose of helping MTs transcribe quickly and accurately, and access to other MTs who just might have the answer. To earn your MT detective badge, you must learn what the best of these resources are and master their use.

Filling in the Blanks, Step by Step

When a dictator says something incomprehensible, the MT inserts a place-holder — or blank — where the mystery word or phrase occurs. Don't be shocked when your transcriptions end up splattered with them, because, especially when you're starting out, they almost certainly will. The good news is that most of them are entirely fixable using the steps in this section.

Many dictators seem to give some thought to the person at the other end of the recording and to what's involved in converting their stream of description into clear patient records and dictate accordingly. Others either don't understand the importance of clear dictation or simply aren't able to accomplish it due to a language barrier or speech impediment. Unfortunately, there aren't just a few difficult dictators; there are many of them.

Even when a dictator speaks clearly, he'll often use highly technical language. Sometimes he may dictate under adverse conditions — in a noisy environment with monitors beeping and children crying, while stuffing down dinner in a few minutes between patients, or while tooling down the highway in a convertible with the top down. At first, it can seem impossible to decipher the dictator's words, but if you follow the steps in this section, before long you'll amaze yourself and others with what you can accurately decipher.

When struggling with difficult dictation, consider this: Terrible dictators offer you job security because no voice-recognition software on earth will ever be able to accurately transcribe their words!

Trust the process

First transcriptions can start out with more holes than a fishing net. It's startlingly common for a new MT to get frustrated to the point of tears due to an inability to decipher what the dictator is saying. You may feel like a failure and wonder if you've made a horrible mistake in selecting this profession. But don't despair — this is a passing condition!

As you develop your ear for dictation, a lot of what formerly sounded like gibberish will

suddenly sound clear. Until (and after) that happens, you can apply some tried-and-true techniques for making those nasty blanks go away.

Remember: As voice recognition technology improves, the difficulty level of dictation MTs must transcribe will increase; the easy stuff will be done by computers. Prepare yourself by becoming an expert at filling in the blanks.

Step 1: Play with the controls

Thank goodness transcription systems come with controls that allow you to adjust playback speed and volume. Be sure to use them! When it comes to speed talkers and mumblers, try slowing things down and turning up the volume. Surprisingly, sometimes actually speeding up the playback speed can make the indistinguishable distinguishable. If you're still having trouble, try unplugging your headphones and listening through your computer speakers instead.

Step 2: Leave it blank (for now)

As counterintuitive as it may feel, the first and often most successful strategy toward resolving a blank is to put in a place holder and keep going. By the time you reach the end of the report, you'll likely know exactly what to put in that spot. Dictators often repeat the same word in different sections of the report, and one of those times — shazam! — you'll realize exactly what it is.

The second thing that makes this strategy work so well is that the first time through a new report, as you're typing it, you naturally tend to focus on words and phrases in pieces. If you listen to the problem section a second time with your transcription in front of you, you'll be more likely to hear whole sentences. When heard in the context of the entire sentence, the mystery word may reveal its true identity.

From a psychological perspective, leaving blanks is not an easy thing for an MT to do. You want to figure out that word or phrase right now! After you've applied this strategy a few times, however, you'll realize it's one of the most effective strategies for filling in blanks.

Step 3: Consider the context

Often, you'll be able to discern a mystery mumbling by considering the words around it. For example, if you think the word is probably the name of a drug, then pay attention to the symptoms and diagnoses of the patient, and the drug name may suddenly leap out at you, especially if it's something common like Lantus insulin for a diabetic.

Thinking about the types of things that typically appear in report sections similar to the one you're typing also can help. In a string of lab results, for example, certain values almost always are grouped together, although not necessarily in the same order. So, if you initially hear, "sodium 141, potassium 3.7, _____ 106," and you know that sodium, potassium, and chloride values typically are grouped together, then most likely chloride is the missing word. This is especially true if you know (or look up) that 106 is a reasonable value for chloride. Listen again with these things in mind and the word *chloride* will likely pop right out.

Anatomy terms are another place where considering surrounding words can help a lot. When you're studying to become an MT, you may wonder why so much emphasis is placed on learning even obscure body parts. After all, the doctor is the medical expert, and you're just transcribing her words, right? If you know your anatomy, when an orthopedist launches into the description of a patient's injury and you hear a phrase that sounds like "fifth meta-something-geal joint," you'll know that if the procedure involves the hand, the word is metacarpophalangeal; if it's the foot, it's metatarsophalangeal. Similarly, the peroneum and perineum are located in quite different places on the human body; if you know anatomy, you'll be able to tell which word the doctor is using.

Step 4: Refer to previous reports

Previous reports by the same dictator can go a long way in helping you sleuth out a tricky bit of dictation. Humans (including dictators) are creatures of habit. When it comes to dictators, this means they tend to dictate certain sections of a report exactly the same way every time (if not identically so, then pretty darn close). This can be very convenient for the MT. For example, a physician may start a review of systems with "No nausea, vomiting, diarrhea, constipation, melena, hemoptysis, hematemesis, cough, or sputum production" every single time, except when there is a notable variation in the particular patient. Get it once, file it away, and you have it forever going forward.

Although looking at previous reports by the same dictator can be incredibly helpful, sometimes you won't have access to them. In such cases, the next best thing is to review reports dictated by other physicians on the same topic. If you're transcribing a C-section and the surgeon says something that sounds like, "A something-steel incision was made with the scalpel and carried down to the fascia," review of another C-section report will quickly identify the garbled word as Pfannenstiel.

Step 5: When in doubt, leave it out

Don't take chances. If you can't confidently fill in a missing word or phrase, leave it blank and flag it for review in whatever manner the rules for the account you're working on specify. A more senior transcriptionist with additional resources to draw on may be able to fill it in. Or the dictator may have to decode her own words, perhaps leading her to dictate more clearly the next time.

Understanding Heavy Accents

Any strong accent, be it East Indian or East Bronx, can present an obstacle to understanding; however, when MTs lament incomprehensible accents, they're typically referring to non-native English speakers, also known as English as a second language (ESL) dictators.

MTs who gripe about ESLs aren't doing so out of impatience or insensitivity — they're doing it because of simple economics. Transcribing a report by an ESL dictator can easily consume double or triple the amount of time as a similar report dictated by a native English speaker. The effect is magnified because the MT fears making mistakes due to difficulty in understanding. This can kill your line count, which, in turn, tanks your paycheck. Get a few ESLs in a row, and it can become understandingly upsetting. If you work on hospital accounts, 40 percent or more of your dictators may be ESL dictators.

To be fair, there are many ESL dictators who far outstrip their native English counterparts in dictation skills. They speak slowly and clearly and enunciate every syllable. Even if they occasionally botch a subject-verb agreement or switch a gender pronoun, they're still great to transcribe for.

However, there are also many ESL dictators who are so difficult to understand that you may question if it's even possible. But unless you're prepared to sharply limit your MT career options, you're going to have to get over it, sharpen your ESL skills, and perhaps even become an ESL specialist.

Relax and then dive in

MTs with little experience transcribing foreign dictators actually may panic a little bit on encountering one in their job queue. This mental tensing up from the expectation of negative consequences has an eerie way of making the very things you fear happen! So, first of all, relax, take a deep breath, and then dive in.

The dictator at the other end of your earphones isn't trying to make your life difficult. In fact, he's probably well aware of — and possibly even self-conscious about — his imperfect English and striving to be as understandable as possible. He's working at his job just as hard as you are, only he has to do it in a non-native language and wrapped in a different culture. A foreign dictator may speak at a barely audible volume because, in his home culture, speaking loudly and assertively is considered rude. He may refer to an object as "he" or "she" because where he grew up, objects have genders.

Instead of avoiding difficult dictators, try to get as many reports by that same dictator as you can lay your hands on in a short period of time. This approach is incredibly effective in helping you develop an ear for a particular accent and speaking style.

Common tendencies of ESL dictators

A dictator's native language uniquely impacts her English pronunciation and grammar, so no single set of rules applies to all cases. However, here are some common characteristics you're likely to encounter:

- ✔ **Dictating punctuation:** Most (though certainly not all) American dictators assume the transcriptionist will insert the proper punctuation in a sentence. An ESL dictator, however, may specify it, even ending a sentence with the word *period* or *full stop.* If you don't realize that's what's happening, you may struggle to figure out what that last word is, when really it's just punctuation.

- ✔ **Sound substitutions:** Letters and sounds that are present in one language may not exist in another. When that happens, a foreign dictator often will swap out the sound with the closest one she knows. The exact substitutions vary by culture, but common swaps include those listed in Table 7-1.

- ✔ **Dropping or adding word endings:** In some cases, the dictator may drop the final letter or syllable of a word entirely or add one on. For example, he may use *fine* instead of *find, chest-ah* instead of *chest,* or *eh-stop* for *stop.*

Table 7-1	Common Sound Substitutions
Problem Sound	*Typical Replacement*
sh (she, sheet)	ch (chee, cheet)
th (this, these, catheter)	D, T, or Z (dis/tis, dees/zees, cadeter)
G or J (gentleman, just)	Y (yentleman, yust)
W (wound, white)	V (vound, vite)
V (virus, Vicryl)	B or W (birus/wirus, Bicryl/Wicryl)
L (collect)	R (correct)

- ✔ **Mixing genders, tenses, and subject-verb agreement:** If an ESL dictator clearly states the patient is a male or female and then seems to randomly apply *he/she* and *him/her* pronouns thereafter, just fix it. The same rule applies for misplaced past/present substitutions and erroneous subject-verb agreements, but only if you're absolutely certain of the correction.

- ✔ **Extra sounds and pauses:** It's common for ESL dictators to insert pauses and interjections *(eh, ah)* while they consider the English words to speak next. If you can't figure out a word the dictator is saying, consider whether it may be one of these.

- ✔ **Misordered words:** If the intent is crystal clear, just reorder it. "The patient tolerated well the procedure" becomes "The patient tolerated the procedure well."

When you "get" a particular ESL dictator, his reports actually can be quicker to transcribe than those of a native English speaker. Because of ESL dictators' more limited English vocabulary, they often rely on set phrasing for everything except non-routine findings. When you know that phrasing, you'll be able to whip through large parts of the report. What you once feared now becomes a benefit.

Virtually all MT jobs today either request or require skill transcribing ESL dictators. Avoid them, and you'll have a hard time finding employment. Embrace them, and you'll be one of the more valuable MTs in the field.

Chapter 8

Mastering the Key Medical Transcription References

In This Chapter

▶ Selecting the best reference resources

▶ Researching medical words and phrases

▶ Digging up laboratory and medication details

*E*ven the most experienced medical transcriptionists (MTs) have to look things up. Knowing where and how to quickly find obscure terms or unfamiliar phrases is a crucial skill that can make the difference between struggling or thriving as an MT.

Information you'll have to look up sooner or later (and often both) includes

✔ Medical words and phrases you haven't heard before

✔ Names of medical and surgical equipment and supplies

✔ Medical abbreviations and acronyms

✔ Brand and generic drug names and dosages

✔ Laboratory tests and normal values

✔ How to format a phrase or document to conform to medical transcription standards

Specialized references exist for every one of these tasks. Some of these are specifically created and designed to make an MT's job easier; others are created for medical professionals or laypeople but are helpful to MTs as well. As your career progresses, you'll develop a customized go-to reference list of your own keyed to the types of reports you transcribe and your personal preferences.

Considering the Source

Whether you go with an electronic resource or a print resource will depend on what's available to you and the task at hand. Websites, spell checkers, and digital references are a boon to MTs, but print books are still sometimes the best go-to resource for looking something up.

For spell checking, an electronic medical spell checker wins hands down over a print medical dictionary. When it comes to figuring out which of the virtually endless variety of forceps a doctor has just named and how to spell it, flipping through the forceps section of a specialty book such as *Stedman's Medical & Surgical Equipment Words* is hard to beat.

Many new MTs make the mistake of heading straight for a search engine when an unfamiliar phrase comes through the headphones, typing in the part they can make out, and hoping to find a website that will fill in the rest. It can work, but it's potentially hazardous.

The treasure trove of information search engines make accessible through a few taps on the keyboard also can be a trap. Those first keystrokes often lead to a few more keystrokes, then 5 minutes, then 30 minutes of perusing before finding a sought-after answer. That's time down the drain. Even worse, the answer may be flat out wrong.

Search engines don't judge the accuracy of a website's content. If you happen to land on a site with inaccurate information and don't realize it, you risk contracting GIGO (garbage in, garbage out) syndrome, something you could pass on to an unfortunate patient by infusing incorrect information into his medical record.

Don't count on Google or another search engine to do your research for you. Search engines can be powerful allies, but only turn to them when you don't have a trusted reference — web-based or otherwise — already at hand.

No single reference tool will solve all your mystery items, but here are the five primary resources MTs rely on to quickly hunt down a mystery word or phrase or verify a word spelling:

- ✔ **Electronic medical spell checkers:** These are simply a must-have for automatic spell checking of medical documents. Stedman's Plus Medical/Pharmaceutical Spellchecker can't be beat for this.

- ✔ **Print and electronic medical dictionaries:** These are useful for checking definitions to ensure that you transcribe exactly the right word, finding the other half of a compound word, looking up Latin terms, getting help with medical prefixes and suffixes, and looking up anatomical terms.

✔ **Specialty word and phrase books designed specifically for medical transcriptionists:** These are useful for deciphering unclear parts of medical words and phrases, spelling words you can essentially understand but have no hope of spelling correctly, and defining acronyms.

✔ **Websites and search engines:** Use these to find physician and medical facility names; define acronyms; and research drug names and doses, lab tests and values, and new-to-market medical devices.

✔ **Fellow MTs:** Turn to your colleagues when all else fails.

Frequently just one of these will suffice, but occasionally you'll have to consult multiple references to confirm your conclusion.

Certain publishers and series have a proven track record of creating excellent medical references. Among them are the following:

✔ The Stedman's series of medical references published by Lippincott, Williams & Wilkins are of the top options on any medical subject.

✔ Saunders, an imprint of Elsevier, publishes specialty books designed for, and often authored by, medical transcriptionists.

✔ The Association for Healthcare Documentation Integrity (AHDI) industry association publishes the standard transcription style guide used by MTs and medical transcription certification exam preparation guides.

✔ Health Professions Institute (HPI) specializes in medical transcription training materials.

Tracking Down Medical Words and Phrases

The first step to hunting down a mystery word or phrase is to assess the surrounding dictation for clues as to what type of word or phrase you're looking for.

✔ What report type and section heading does it appear under?

✔ Is it linked to a particular specialty (for example, cardiology, obstetrics, orthopedics)?

✔ Is it related to a body part or system?

✔ What part of speech is it (noun, adjective, verb, and so on)?

✔ Could it be a piece of medical equipment or a drug name?

✔ Could it be an acronym pronounced as a word? (For example, CABG is frequently dictated as "cabbage.")

Use the answers to select the best reference for the job.

You may be tempted to let medical spell checkers help you find the right word for you or warn you if you've typed the wrong one, but don't do it! They only check if you've typed a correctly spelled word, not whether it's the *right* word. It's up to you to know (or research) the difference between *mucus* and *mucous* or soundalike drug names such as clonidine and Klonopin.

Beyond definitions: Mining a medical dictionary

Medical dictionaries offer a lot more than a way to look up a definition or spelling of a word that you already know; they also help you find multipart words and phrases when you can recognize one part of it but not the other.

There are two commercial (not free) medical dictionaries MTs frequently use:

✔ *Stedman's Medical Dictionary,* published by Lippincott, Williams & Wilkins

✔ *Dorland's Illustrated Medical Dictionary,* published by Elsevier Saunders

You only need one or the other, not both. Available in print and electronic versions, they're packed with features that are very useful to MTs. In addition to detailed definitions, they include

✔ Subentries under each noun, listing adjectives and eponyms related to it

✔ Special sections like Word Finder and Genus Finder that provide alternate ways to look things up

✔ Illustrations that identify anatomical parts and concepts

The first two features are incredibly helpful for pinning down partial words and phrases. For example, if a dictator is describing a hand injury and says "Bennett fracture," but all you can make out is "ben___ fracture," whip out your medical dictionary, open it to the "fracture" entry in the main A-to-Z section, and scan down the subentries beneath it. There it is: Bennett fracture, a fracture dislocation of the thumb. Puzzle solved! Figure 8-1 shows the subentries for the word Fracture in *Dorland's Illustrated Medical Dictionary*, 32nd Edition.

Figure 8-1:
Fracture
listing from
*Dorland's
Illustrated
Medical
Dictionary.*

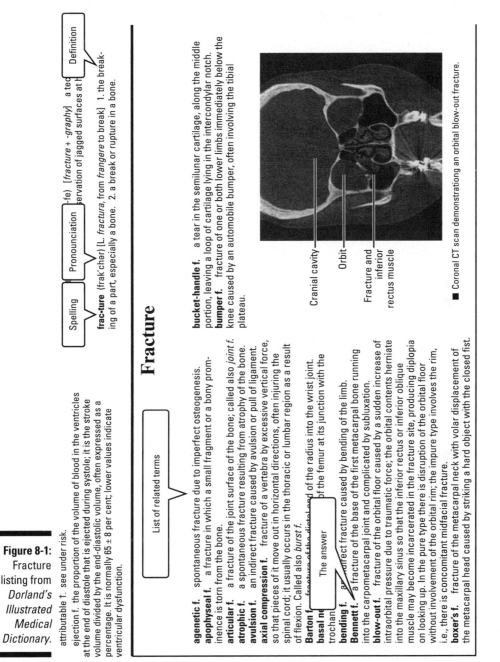

| Spelling | Pronunciation | Definition |

frac·ture (frak'chər) [*fracture* + *-graphy*] a tec...servation of jagged surfaces at... 1. the break-ing of a part, especially a bone. 2. a break or rupture in a bone.

attributable t. see under risk.
ejection f. the proportion of the volume of blood in the ventricles at the end of diastole that is ejected during systole; it is the stroke volume divided by the end-diastolic volume, often expressed as a percentage. It is normally 65 ± 8 per cent; lower values indicate ventricular dysfunction.

List of related terms

The answer

Fracture

agenetic f. spontaneous fracture due to imperfect osteogenesis.
apophyseal f. a fracture in which a small fragment or a bony prominence is torn from the bone.
articular f. a fracture of the joint surface of the bone; called also *joint f.*
atrophic f. a spontaneous fracture resulting from atrophy of the bone.
avulsion f. an indirect fracture caused by avulsion or pull of ligament.
axial compression f. fracture of a vertebra by excessive vertical force, so that pieces of it move out in horizontal directions, often injuring the spinal cord; it usually occurs in the thoracic or lumbar region as a result of flexion. Called also *burst f.*
Barton f. fracture of the distal end of the radius into the wrist joint.
basal n...of the femur at its junction with the trochan...
bending f. an indirect fracture caused by bending of the limb.
Bennett f. a fracture of the base of the first metacarpal bone running into the carpometacarpal joint and complicated by subluxation.
blow-out f. fracture of the orbital floor caused by a sudden increase of intraorbital pressure due to traumatic force; the orbital contents herniate into the maxillary sinus so that the inferior rectus or inferior oblique muscle may become incarcerated in the fracture site, producing diplopia on looking up. In the pure type there is disruption of the orbital floor without involvement of the orbital rim; the impure type involves the rim, i.e., there is concomitant midfacial fracture.
boxer's f. fracture of the metacarpal neck with volar displacement of the metacarpal head caused by striking a hard object with the closed fist.

bucket-handle f. a tear in the semilunar cartilage, along the middle portion, leaving a loop of cartilage lying in the intercondylar notch.
bumper f. fracture of one or both lower limbs immediately below the knee caused by an automobile bumper, often involving the tibial plateau.

Cranial cavity

Orbit

Fracture and
inferior
rectus muscle

■ Coronal CT scan demonstrating an orbital blow-out fracture.

What if you're pretty sure the first word is "Bennett," but you're not clear what comes after that? Either look up Bennett in the A-to-Z listings, or jump to the Word Finder section and look for it there. Remember to try alternate spellings (such as "Bennit" or "Benett") if you don't hit it the first time.

The A-to-Z entry for Bennett, shown in Figure 8-2, will inform you that Bennett is a name, and that it is associated with the word "fracture." This information alone may be enough to solve your mystery, but if not, follow the trail provided to the "see under *fracture*" reference.

Figure 8-2:
The Bennett
A-to-Z
Listing from
*Dorland's
Illustrated
Medical
Dictionary*
reveals that
Bennett is
the name
of an Irish
surgeon.

be•nign (bə-nīn´) [L. *benignus*] not malignant; not recurrent; favorable for recovery.

be•nig•nan•cy (bə-nig´nan-se″) the quality of being benign.

Ben•nett fracture (ben´et) [Edward Hallaran *Bennett*, Irish surgeon, 1837–1907] see under *fracture.*

Ben•o•quin (ben´o-kwin) trademark for preparations of monobenzone.

ben•ox•i•nate hy•dro•chlo•ride (ben-ok´sĭ-nāt) [USP] a benzoic acid ester related to procaine, used as a topical anesthetic in ophthalmology; applied topically to the conjunctiva to produce anesthesia of short duration.

This dictionary listing was published in Dorland's Illustrated Medical Dictionary, 32nd edition, Page 208, Copyright Saunders, an Imprint of Elsevier, Inc. (2012).

The illustrations in a medical dictionary come in handy when you're transcribing a report and a doctor names an unfamiliar or barely comprehensible anatomical feature. If you know the body part (for example, the hip), you can look for a corresponding anatomical diagram in the dictionary, and it will often identify every organ, bone, nerve, muscle, tissue, and vessel in that area, along with their sub-parts.

The figures used in the previous examples are from a print medical dictionary, but the same features are available in the electronic versions (see the nearby sidebar for more).

Every time you obtain a new reference, invest a few minutes to read the introductory material describing how best to use it. You'll almost always discover time-saving features and techniques you otherwise would miss out on.

Just OneLook

A favorite (and, coincidentally, free) online dictionary resource is OneLook (www.onelook. com). It has a simple, easy-to-use interface and searches multiple dictionaries with a single click. You also can search using word patterns, which means you can find words you aren't sure how to spell. The results page displays matching words it found and where it found them. You can click on any result that looks promising to go to the original source and view the full definition.

By default, OneLook searches all dictionaries in its database, not just medical dictionaries; however, you can direct it to show results from medical dictionaries first by adjusting the settings available through the "Customize" link at the top of the home page. You also can control other features, including whether definitions are opened in the same browser window or in a new one and how much detail is included in the search results.

Although it's a popular MT research tool, OneLook is not designed specifically for medical users and has shortcomings to keep in mind. Because it's a search engine, remember to assess the sources of the results it provides before using them, and pay close attention to the capitalization and formatting of any results you decide to use.

Medical word books

Medical word books, which come in print and electronic versions, are lists of words and short phrases organized in alphabetical order. Their sole purpose is to help you speedily locate words and phrases and spell them correctly, and they do it well. They don't include definitions, so if you're unsure you have the right word, you'll need to check with a resource that does.

Medical word books come in two flavors:

✔ **General purpose:** The general-purpose books are designed for width and throw in everything but the kitchen sink into one large reference. Although that may sound very convenient, in reality it's quite limiting because depth into individual medical word categories is sacrificed to achieve greater scope.

✔ **Specialty:** The specialty books, on the other hand, bypass the big picture in favor of depth on a single topic or a pair of closely intertwined topics, for example:

• Single medical specialty area (orthopedics, oncology, general surgery, and so on)

• Medical word category that is applicable to multiple specialties (for example, medical equipment, laboratory terms, or radiology words)

> Specialty books cram a whole lot of words into a compact, focused reference, and go much deeper into the terminology of the topic than either dictionaries or general medical word books do.

Both types of word books contain multiple listings for a phrase — often one under each word in the phrase. If you can get a word or two of a short phrase, you often can use a medical word book to quickly and definitively identify the full phrase.

For example, imagine you're transcribing a cardiology consultation, and the patient is diagnosed with "inferior walrus infarction." Huh? You replay it again and hear the same thing. If you have a cardiology specialty word book such as *Stedman's Cardiovascular & Pulmonary Words* on hand, you can consult it and quickly resolve your confusion:

1. Look up *infarction,* and you'll find *inferior wall infarction.*
2. Look up inferior, and you'll find inferior wall infarction.
3. Look up *walrus,* and you'll find . . . nothing, of course!

You also can resolve this using a general word book, but it would be more challenging. In the general word book, you'd find pages and pages of infarction-related words; because infarctions aren't limited to the heart, they also occur in other organs, including the brain, kidney, eye, and even placenta.

There are specialty word books covering virtually every medical topic an MT may encounter, but rest assured you don't need them all! You only need those that closely correlate to the reports you most frequently transcribe.

If you transcribe any acute-care reports, a medical and surgical equipment word book is invaluable. For starters, there are more than 3,500 different forceps, and catheters come in over 2,000 varieties. A doctor never grasps with forceps or places a catheter; she grasps with Luikart-Kjelland obstetrical forceps or places a Swan-Ganz thermodilution catheter. If you can spell those without looking them up, there may be a place for you in *The Guinness Book of World Records.*

Abbreviation and acronym finders

In order to produce the clearest medical document possible, MTs expand acronyms, abbreviations, and other verbal shortcuts to eliminate misinterpretation of their meaning.

WARNING!

Many acronyms have multiple potential expansions. If you're not absolutely certain you've found the right one, don't expand it!

The best way to look these is up is to use a specialty book or trusted website that specializes in medical acronyms. The number-one option is *Stedman's Abbreviations, Acronyms & Symbols.* Another reference, less comprehensive and focused but still useful, is AcronymFinder.com (`www.acronymfinder.com`).

If you have a specialty medical word book that covers the relevant specialty or word category, that's another great place to look.

TECHNICAL STUFF

Conducting a fuzzy search

What can you do when you need to look up something, but you're a little fuzzy on the exact wording or spelling? Turn to a search tool that's fuzzy, too, naturally. Feed it a few wildcards, and you're off and running.

Fuzzy searches use pattern matching to find near matches in addition to exact matches. Many searches automatically go fuzzy to a very limited extent — if nothing exactly matches the terms you entered, they'll look into a private "oops" file of common typos and misspellings and try to guess what you probably meant to type rather than what you did. That's helpful, but there's a lot more power available through judicious use of wildcards.

Wildcards are special characters that serve as placeholders. When you add a wildcard to your search query, you're essentially inserting a blank you want the search engine to fill in. The two wildcards you need to know are ? (question mark) and * (asterisk). The ? is equivalent to a blank exactly one character wide. Although you can use more than one ? in a query, it's still not terribly useful unless you know almost exactly what you're searching for. The * (asterisk), on the other hand, inserts a blank big enough to hold an entire string of characters, making it much more versatile.

Here are some example searches:

✔ **opt?c:** Finds words that start with *opt,* end with *c,* and have one character in between

✔ **opt*:** Finds words and phrases that start with *opt*

✔ ***opt:** Finds words and phrases that end with *opt*

✔ **opt*opt:** Finds words and phrases that start and end with *opt*

There's a critical difference between the major online search engines and stand-alone electronic references such as the kind you might install on your computer. Although the electronic references allow you to use an asterisk wildcard at the beginning, end, or middle of a character string, major search engines, including Google and Bing, do not. They treat the asterisk as a placeholder for one or more words, not one or more characters. So, the asterisk must have a space on either side and shouldn't abut against anything. Thus, what you might enter as *inferior w* infarct* into most electronic searches should be entered as *inferior * infarct* to get the desired results in Google or Bing.

Nailing Down Drugs and Dosages

Transcribing medications correctly is absolutely critical. Most dictators take special care to be clear when dictating a medication list, but there are still plenty of occasions when you'll have to use references to clear up murky spots.

Top drug references for medical transcriptionists

Favorite MT resources for researching medications include the following:

✔ *Quick Look Drug Book* **(QLDB), by Leonard L. Lance (Lippincott Williams & Wilkins):** The electronic version (it's also available as a printed book) of the QLDB offers the most versatile way to find and verify drug names and dosages. You can use fuzzy searches, look up medications by drug class/medical condition, find brand-name versions of generic drugs and vice versa, and check common dosages. You can add custom comments to any entry, and in the rare case that a drug you're looking for is not in the QLDB, you can add it yourself for future use. Because it's designed for quick lookups, you won't have to plow through extra information that's not relevant to your needs. You'll have to purchase a license to use the QLDB, but it's well worth the investment.

✔ **Drugs.com** (www.drugs.com)**:** This free website offers a quick way to look up drug names, dosage formats, and the conditions the drug is prescribed for. You can search by brand or generic drug name or browse an alphabetical list. One of the best features is the ability to conduct a phonetic search. Type in what the drug name sounds like, and Drugs.com will search for medications with a similar pronunciation. Type in *rantedeen* and up pops *ranitidine*. You also can do wildcard searches. Drugs.com has the major plus of being free and available from anywhere that has an Internet connection. On the downside, it's not as succinct as the QLDB, and you'll have to scan through extra material to get to the information you need.

✔ *Physician's Desk Reference* **(PDR):** The PDR is a comprehensive prescribing reference that's on hand in virtually all medical offices. I include it in this list primarily because it's so well known that most MTs are aware of it even if they don't choose to use it. If you're working on-site at a physician's office or hospital, you may receive free access to the PDR. It offers multiple ways to look up drugs and dosages, and you can count on it being accurate and thorough. It includes much more intensive detail than the other resources, though, which can be a drawback when you just want to confirm spelling or dosage options.

Clearing up cloudy medication details

Drugs are frequently dictated as lists. An individual drug typically consists of up to five parts. Use the segments you hear clearly to help track down the parts you're unsure of.

Drug Name	Dosage	Dosage Format	Quantity	Administration Route	Frequency
atenolol	50 mg	tablets	One	p.o.	b.i.d.

Although this is the standard format, a dictator may not include all the segments, or she may include them in a different order. Thus, if you hear:

> atenolol 50 milligrams one __ b.i.d.

It's likely the mystery word describes either the dosage format or the administration route. Listen again for "tablet," "by mouth" or "p.o."

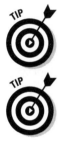

If the dictator is dictating a list of medications, he tends to stick to the same format for all of them. Use the medication items you can understand to determine the order and segments this particular dictator uses, and that will help you identify which segment the part that you're trying to figure out most likely belongs to.

Here are some additional strategies

✔ **If you can't make out a drug name:** Use a fuzzy search to put in your best guess and see what turns up. Compare the results to the patient's condition(s) to find the most likely match. If you can make out the dictated dosage amount, format, and/or administration route, eliminate any results that aren't available in forms that meet those criteria. Then listen again to determine if you can now identify what the dictator is naming.

As an alternative, use a reference that allows you to list drugs by medical condition. Scan it for the closest matches and then follow the preceding steps.

✔ **If you're unclear on the drug dosage amount or frequency or administration segments (for example, you're not sure if the dictator said 15 or 50 mg tablets):** Look up the drug name and check the available dosages (does it come in 15 mg or 50 mg tablets?), available formats (tablets, syrup, Dosepak, Respules), and recommended dosing ranges.

Keep in mind that there are many drugs with similar-sounding names, so be alert to mismatches between medication and the patient's condition or the dictated dosage and the standard dosage range used for that drug.

Dictators occasionally make mistakes when dictating drug names and dosages. If something seems awry, research it. If it still seems doubtful, don't hesitate to flag it and bring it to the dictator's attention for clarification.

Checking Up on Laboratory Tests

The easy part of transcribing laboratory values is that it's usually obvious when a dictator is listing test results; the hard part is that they often get spit out in one long sentence, and it's not always a clear one. Fortunately, lab values almost always are grouped together based on the type of test. Identify the test group, and you're well on your way to resolving any unclear spots.

For example, one of the most commonly ordered blood tests is the complete blood count (CBC). CBC results include values for white blood cells (WBCs), red blood cells (RBCs), hemoglobin, and hematocrit. The results are dictated as name/value pairs (WBCs 8000, RBCs 5.1).

To check up on lab dictation you're unsure of, follow these steps:

1. **Identify the name of the test group the result most likely belongs to, such as blood count, thyroid panel, or coagulation profile.**

   If you're not familiar with the group, a search for lab tests related to the conditions the patient has may turn it up.

2. **Determine which values in that group you haven't yet transcribed.**

   These are your prime candidates.

3. **Look up the test group in your reference and scan through the name/ value pairs it typically includes to see if your mystery item is present.**

   Pay particular attention to the normal results range of that test and the value you think you hear to be sure they correlate.

As you gain experience, you'll type the same lab result groups again and again. Before long, you'll almost instantly know what should come next and even notice when a dictated value is out of whack.

Favorite MT references for identifying and confirming laboratory test names and expected normal values include the following:

✔ **Lab Tests Online** (www.labtestsonline.org)**:** This free resource is great for identifying lab tests by formal or informal name or by medical condition. It's not much use for checking reference ranges, however.

✔ **Wikipedia's Reference ranges for blood tests entry** (`http://en.wikipedia.org/wiki/Reference_ranges_for_common_blood_tests`): This page includes an extensive list of reference ranges for blood tests. It also links to reference ranges for additional lab test types, such as urinalyses.

Appendix B lists common lab test groups and provides examples of transcribed lab results.

Consulting the Book (of Style)

Applying standard formatting and punctuation is a core part of your job as an MT, but there are so many rules, it's virtually impossible to keep track of them all, especially when starting out. Fortunately there's a reference dedicated to keeping track of the rules for you.

The Book of Style for Medical Transcription (BOS for short), which is published by the Association for Healthcare Documentation Integrity (AHDI), is the widely accepted arbiter of medical document formatting. You should always follow it, with one exception: if your employer specifies otherwise.

Transcription accounts may have in-house standards that vary from what AHDI recommends. Account specifics always take priority over *The Book of Style.*

Calling on Colleagues for Help

Your reference of last resort is fellow MTs. Why last? Because although MTs are frequently willing to help each other out, to do so they must put their own production on pause. Most MT positions tightly link pay to lines transcribed, so unless the person you ask for help is your supervisor (and sometimes even then), any time she spends helping you is essentially unpaid.

When you're just starting out, you're going to have to get help from your supervisor and other MTs. There's just no way around it, and they (and you) should expect that and not be distressed by it. After you make it past the newbie stage, you should be able to solve all but the most vexing transcription challenges on your own. With your favorite references at your fingertips and the know-how to use them, you'll be able to offer help rather than request it.

Dictations gone witty: True tales from the trenches

You never know what may come over the headphones — at times, it can trigger giggles or a quick "get this!" e-mail to an MT friend. The following quotes are drawn verbatim from transcription recordings; they're things dictators actually said, or at least what the transcriptionists think they said:

- ✔ "The patient unfortunately has gained a little bit of weight since last time, but he went through the trauma of having to eat through his birthday desserts."

- ✔ "John states his girlfriend has noted he seems to be breathing heavier at times. Of note, his girlfriend is now pregnant."

- ✔ "This is a 63-year-old male, I believe he is homeless, who was brought to the emergency by the paramedics after someone called 911 to his house."

- ✔ "The patient denies any foul smell to the diarrhea."

- ✔ "She is asking for a pill for her nastiness."

- ✔ "The patient's name is 539007."

- ✔ "He will have nurse therapy as well."

- ✔ "Typically, the headache seems to radiate to the head."

- ✔ "It is obvious that the patient drinks. I am unaware of any drug abuse or drinking."

- ✔ "The baby was present at birth."

- ✔ "The patient has a history of sudden death."

Chapter 9

Meeting the Need for Speed

*W*hen it comes to medical transcription, time = money, plain and simple. To make money doing medical transcription, you simply have to transcribe quickly. No matter how fast you can type and reference, you won't realize your true income potential until you start leveraging the power of technology. You can easily double or triple your productivity (and income) by employing the techno tools and techniques in this chapter. If you don't care how much you earn, go ahead and skip this chapter; otherwise, get ready to start your journey to Master of Faster.

The art and science of transcribing faster has three underlying key principles:

✔ Keep your hands on the keyboard as much as possible. Don't reach for that mouse or trackball if you can accomplish the same task with a keyboard shortcut.

✔ Dig deep into productivity software, and learn everything you can about it.

✔ Set up your computer with speed in mind (but don't sacrifice ergonomics, or you won't be speedy for very long).

In this chapter, you explore the incredible super powers word expanders bring to your fingertips and why mastering them, not just using them, pays off. You also meet macros, which allow you to execute an entire string of actions with one or two keystrokes. Last, you find out how easy it is to attach a second monitor to your computer and why you may want to do so.

When you first try a new productivity tool, your line count may actually drop temporarily, but stick with it and have faith: It's a trend that will quickly reverse. When you get through the initial learning curve, speed will come your way, and lots of it. You can use it to earn a substantially larger paycheck or to reduce the hours you need to put in to meet a line production goal — it's up to you.

Mastering the Number-One Speed Tool: Word Expanders

A *word expander* (also known as a *text expander*) is a bit of software wizardry that sits in the background, monitoring what you type. When you enter a letter combination you've previous identified as a shortcut, the system replaces it with the full monty — on the fly. For example, you type

> tp

and hit the spacebar. Before you can blink, the word expander swoops in and replaces it with

> the patient

You put in 2 characters and got 11 out, what a deal! Your output just more than quintupled! Shortcuts can be created for anything from a single word to entire blocks of text. *Every keystroke you save is money in your pocket.* Here's a longer example:

Without a word expander:

> The patient is a 29-year-old white female who has a history of

With a word expander (a savings of 43 characters):

> tpia 29 yo wf whaho

Things you can do with a word expander besides expand words

You can use word expanders to do a lot more than just expand words and phrases. Really they should be called "swappers" instead of expanders. You can create shortcuts that

✔ Eliminate the need to reach for awkward (and slow) key combinations (*vqs* becomes *V/Q scan*)

✔ Remember proper formatting and capitalization for you (*q46h* becomes *q.4-6 h.*)

✔ Fix typos you commonly make (*seh* becomes *she*)

✔ Replace unacceptable abbreviations and slang with approved alternatives (*qd* becomes *daily*)

Remember: An expander determines what to do with a shortcut by looking in a storage file, or glossary, of shortcuts and expansions. You have complete control of what that file contains and can add to or edit it at will.

Don't worry, you won't have to memorize a bunch of cryptic letter combinations like *whaho* to harness the power of word expansion. The shortcut *whaho* is simply the first letter of each word in the phrase *who has a history of*. It's a system. If you know the rules of the system, you know the shortcut — and you're guaranteed to know the rules, because you create them.

Choosing a word expander

There's more than one way to get your hands on a word expander. You can pick one out and buy it yourself (highly recommended) or use one that's provided to you. They come in two forms:

- ✔ **Standalone software applications:** Installing a standalone expander is like adding a utility service to your computer. After you fire it up, it runs in the background, making shortcut functionality available to other programs you use. Standalone expanders aren't always compatible with every possible application you may use, but they're amazingly versatile. They'll work right alongside Microsoft Word and many specialized medical transcription platforms.

- ✔ **Built-in features of other programs:** Expanders that exist as integrated features of other programs are much less versatile. They often come at a great price, though: free. Many medical transcriptionists (MTs) do their transcribing with Microsoft Word. Its AutoCorrect feature is essentially an expander. It has very limited functionally compared to standalone expanders, but you can put it to good use if you understand it well.

Power and portability make a stand-alone the best option for those who get to choose. They aren't free, but your initial investment will pay off many times over, especially if you become an expander master. As an added bonus, if you end up working on a different transcription platform, your shortcuts often can come right along with you. And that's not all . . . if you order today, you can also swap expander files with other MTs who use the same system, if you're so inclined. Two expanders are particularly popular among MTs:

- ✔ Instant Text, by Textware Solutions (www.fitaly.com)
- ✔ Shorthand for Windows by OfficeSoft (www.pcshorthand.com)

Instant Text is more powerful, but both of them have busloads of MT cheerleaders and way too many fabulous features to list here. Fortunately, they also both have fully functional 30-day trial versions, so you can test-drive them and pick a favorite.

If you work on a proprietary medical transcription platform, it may have an expander built in. Just because it's there, however, doesn't necessarily mean it's your only option. Instant Text or Shorthand for Windows may well work with the platform, even if your employer isn't aware of it. Because the stand-alones are usually better, try one out and see what happens.

As an extra incentive, keep in mind that if you're using a built-in expander program and you happen to change employers, you'll most likely have to leave your entire, wonderful expander file behind and start a new one from scratch. If you want to see a seasoned MT cry, take away her word expander. Just make sure you're standing well out of reach first.

Becoming an expander ninja

Expanders are personal. You can customize them to fit how you think, what you particularly like or dislike typing, and the kinds of reports you transcribe. No two MTs use the same expander the same way. The power you get out of your expander has everything to do with what you put into it.

Expander programs come fully functional out of the box, and often even have a generic starter library of shortcuts. However, like training wheels on a bike, that starter library can go from helper to impediment pretty quickly. When you're ready to get serious, you'll need to lose the training wheels. In expander-land, that means tossing that starter file and building a shortcut library that works as you do. So, where do you start?

- **RTFM (read the fabulous manual) that came with your expander.** It won't kill you, and you'll learn amazing tricks your expander can perform that you'd otherwise completely miss out on. Every word expander comes with its own repertoire of cool, productivity-boosting stuff, so it's not a "seen one, seen 'em all" kind of thing. What if it could do the dishes for you if you only knew which keys to press?

- **Start slowly and adapt.** The thrill of quadrupling productivity gets many MTs feverishly adding shortcuts the minute the program is installed. You may get a lot of shortcuts in there fast, but they won't be the right shortcuts. You're better off using the system a bit and trying out different options. There'll be some initial trial and error in discovering what works best for you — that's part of the process of building a killer system. Allow for that time, and your patience will pay off. Then you can start feverishly adding shortcuts.

- **Use a system to determine your shortcuts.** You can't possibly remember the thousand-plus shortcuts you'll eventually have in your files, but you can remember a set of rules. Plus, you don't have to create a system from scratch; those who have expanded before you have blazed trails you can follow. Two of the best places to start:

  - The book *Saving Keystrokes,* by Diana Rolland, is packed with awesome techniques and examples.

  - The ABCZ system (`www.jonknowles.net/abczhome.htm`) created by Jon Knowles is another favorite.

These systems employ very different techniques, but both are very powerful. One will probably resonate with you more than the other. Ultimately, you may decide to devise your own system, but surveying what's already out there first is a good idea. At the very least, you'll get some ideas for techniques you want to borrow or avoid.

Don't wait until you graduate from a training program to get some word expander practice. Yes, it's best to start by typing reports out in full, the old-fashioned way, so you can etch into your mind how various things should be done, but as you near graduation, find a word expander somewhere and start using it.

WARNING! Beware of unintended expansions! Sooner or later it *will* happen: You'll type something you wanted to appear exactly as entered, forgetting you previously used it as a shortcut. Your expander won't forget, and it will do its job and expand it. If you don't notice, the results can be embarrassing. Unwanted expansions also can happen when you back up to correct something and confuse the poor expander.

TIP Every expander program has a "suppression" function. If you don't want a particular combination to expand in a particular instance, you hit the suppression key combination instead of the space key, and you're on your way free and clear (and expansion-less). Want to know which keys to press? You'll have to read the manual, because each expander is different.

REMEMBER Your expander is a pipeline bringing you increased income. Back up that expander file regularly!

Taking Advantage of Macros

A macro is a recording of a series of actions grouped together. You can execute the macro with a single key press or key combination called a *hot key* or *keyboard shortcut.* Macros can prove quite handy for automating tasks you perform frequently.

For example, preoperative and postoperative diagnoses are often the same, so a surgeon may dictate the first diagnoses list and then say "same" for the second. You have three options for handling it:

✔ Add the new heading "Postoperative Diagnoses" and retype the diagnoses individually. This is the slowest and most error-prone method.

✔ Select and copy the preoperative list, and then paste it back into the document and replace the title of the copied version with "Postoperative Diagnoses." This is better than the preceding option, but slower than the next one.

✔ Create a macro that does the copying/pasting for you and assign it a keyboard shortcut, such as Alt+F5. Every time you run across the "same," just hit Alt+F5, let the macro do its handiwork, and you're on your merry way.

The best-known macro maker is the one built into Microsoft Word. Macros that perform basic tasks, like moving around a cursor or cutting and pasting, can be easily created using Word's "Record Macro" feature. More complex macros require programming skills. Because the steps to create a macro vary between versions of Word, the best way to learn the right steps for your version is to fire up Word's Help feature and search for "record macro."

Standalone macro tools bring the power of macros to your entire computer. AutoHotkey (www.autohotkey.com) is free software that allows you to automate almost anything you can do with your keyboard or mouse, not just inside a particular program, but virtually anywhere on a computer that's running Windows. With it, you can get really deep into automating, even creating macros that include muting your sound card, opening and closing individual windows, copying and pasting between programs, and more.

Creating and using macros is substantially more complex than using expander software, but so are the tasks macros can perform. Whether you should use them comes down to your MT needs and how tech-savvy you are. Macros can be helpful, but they aren't essential. Expander software, on the other hand, is essential.

If all this talk about expanders, macros, and shortcut systems has your mind buzzing with questions, head straight to Productivity Talk (www.productivitytalk.com). There, you'll find lots of friendly folks who are experts on all this stuff. It's a great place to discuss the merits of different word expanders, shortcut systems, and macro making. Although it's not just for MTs, many hang out there.

Your Computer on Steroids: Using Dual Monitors

Setting up your computer to use multiple monitors will forever change the way you work with your computer, not only for medical transcription, but for everything else, too. It's very easy to do, even if you're "technically challenged." Once you do it, you'll wonder how you ever got by with one measly monitor for so many years. Figure 9-1 shows what a typical multi-monitor setup looks like.

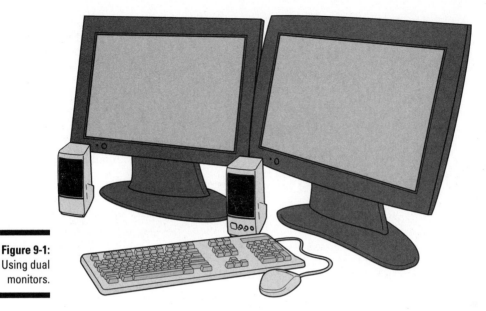

Figure 9-1:
Using dual
monitors.

Why is this such an incredible productivity booster? Consider how many times each day you switch back and forth between a document you're working on and references you're using at the same time. MTs do it constantly, because referencing is a key part of the job. (Perhaps you also check Facebook or e-mail, but we're talking MT productivity here, so we'll pretend you don't do that other stuff during work hours). With a single-monitor setup, you can look at one application or the other, but not both at the same time. With two monitors attached to your computer, you can have both (and potentially more) visible at the same time.

You may think switching between application views is plenty fast already, especially if you the use keyboard shortcut Alt+tab to do it. That sensation of speed is misleading, because every time you flip between screens, your mind has to adjust, too. When you return to the document you're transcribing, you have to find your place and mentally pick up where you left off. You have to do so while holding what you just referenced in your mind. You might sometimes have to go back and look at the reference multiple times. The reality of MT work is that you're paid only for lines you produce, not time you spend referencing, so the quicker you can find what you're looking for and get back to cranking out lines, the better. All that flipping back and forth consumes time and mental energy that could be better spent boosting your paycheck.

By adding a second monitor, you can keep your transcription software always in front of you on the primary monitor and never switch away from it.

Dedicate the second one to referencing, instant messaging your supervisor, and tasks like checking e-mail. No more flipping back and forth on one screen!

Here's what you'll need:

- ✔ A current desktop or laptop computer running a reasonably recent version of Microsoft Windows
- ✔ An additional monitor with cable to connect it to your computer

Microsoft will gladly walk you through dual-monitor setup using various versions of Windows. Just visit this web page: `www.microsoft.com/athome/organization/twomonitors.aspx`.

Usually all you'll have to do is plug your new monitor into an open video connection (a port) on your existing computer, and Microsoft Windows automatically detects and configures the new monitor. Then you can make adjustments regarding how you want the monitors to work. For example, you can opt to treat the two monitors as separate screens or as if they were one continuous screen.

If you want to connect a second monitor to a laptop that has no external video connection port, you can create a monitor connection using a USB port instead. You'll need a VGA to USB conversion cable to pull it off.

The one potential tricky spot is that the new monitor's cable type must be a match for the opening (port) you plan to plug it into. If you're buying a new monitor, make sure you pick one (and the cable to go with it) that's compatible with your computer. Most modern monitors have multiple connection types built in. Of course, your second monitor doesn't have to be modern, it can be a hand-me-down and still work fine. If you end up with a monitor that doesn't have the right kind of connector, you have two options:

- ✔ Attach a video adapter to your computer to change the connection type.
- ✔ Replace your current video card or install an additional video card with the needed connection type.

Even if you have to hire a computer whiz to replace your video card, it's well worth the cost for the productivity you'll gain in return.

Part III

Looking at the Types of Reports You'll Transcribe

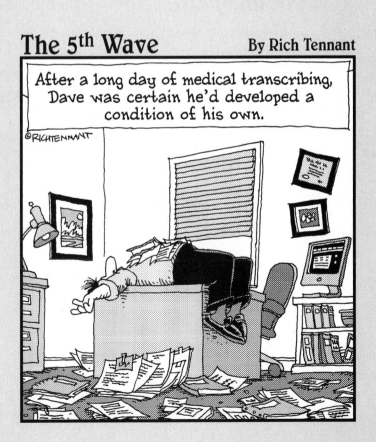

The 5th Wave   By Rich Tennant

After a long day of medical transcribing, Dave was certain he'd developed a condition of his own.

In this part . . .

Introducing the Big Four: the family of reports that comprise the core of medical transcription work. In this part, you step through each of them in detail, including section headings, formatting, and organization. Then it's off to meet the relatives — another half-dozen report types that are likely to cross your desk.

Chapter 10

History and Physical Examination

The admitting History and Physical Examination (known as an H&P) is the flagship of the "Big Four" reports that make up the core of medical transcription work. It's almost as if you're standing beside the healthcare provider as he meets the patient for the first time. If you're like most MTs, it won't be long before you start assessing symptoms, evaluating lab results, and diagnosing the patient yourself, before the official diagnoses are dictated.

An H&P is the first document added to a patient's medical record. It's the intake form used by hospitals, specialty clinics, and physicians seeing a patient for the first time. In an emergency situation, the surgeon needs that H&P in hand by the time a patient reaches the operating room (OR).

An H&P describes the patient's initial symptoms and the history leading up to them, explores potential contributing factors, identifies potential diagnoses, and maps out a starting treatment plan. At its heart lies a detailed physical examination that methodically reviews all major body systems. From its creation onward, the H&P is referred to by all healthcare providers with access to the chart that contains it. On repeat visits, additional reports are generated to document progress, treatments, operations, and so forth, but the initial H&P remains the anchor for the patient record.

In this chapter, I cover all the sections of an H&P that you're likely to find. But first I start with an overview.

For more on formatting reports, turn to Chapter 6.

A sample full H&P report is included in Appendix C.

Overview

The degree of detail included in a History and Physical Examination report is determined by the nature and complexity of a patient's condition. The H&P for a patient with a straightforward, self-limiting problem can be quite brief. Reports on patients with multiple chronic conditions and/or acute illnesses or injuries can go into exhaustive detail.

An initial H&P typically includes the following major sections:

- ✔ **Chief Complaint:** A succinct statement of the patient's current primary problem(s)
- ✔ **History of Present Illness:** A narrative history of precipitating events related to the patient's current status
- ✔ **Past History:** Details of the patient's previous medical conditions and surgeries, family medical history, social history, and personal habits
- ✔ **Allergies:** Whether the patient has any allergies to medications and what they are
- ✔ **Medications:** List of the patient's current medications
- ✔ **Review of Systems:** An inventory of symptoms the patient is currently experiencing, as reported by the patient
- ✔ **Physical Examination:** Objective physical and mental examination findings, often thorough and quite detailed
- ✔ **Diagnostic Studies:** Results of laboratory tests, imaging, EKGs, and other diagnostic evaluations previously performed
- ✔ **Impression:** Analyses of the patient's condition and potential diagnoses
- ✔ **Plan:** The next steps in the patient's treatment

Most, but not all, of the examples in this chapter use heading and layout styles as recommended in *The Book of Style for Medical Transcription*, 3rd Edition, by AHDI. Some of the examples stray *from The Book of Style* in order to demonstrate other common layouts you're likely to encounter, because report formatting varies to some degree between facilities. Dictators don't always word headings identically, though the meaning is still clear, and the examples reflect that as well. When transcribing, you should always format reports and headings as specified by the account you're working on, regardless of what standards might otherwise apply.

The purpose of headings is to organize a report and make it easy to locate specific content. If a dictator starts a section that obviously belongs under a particular heading but doesn't explicitly dictate the heading, it's acceptable practice for the medical transcriptionist (MT) to insert it.

Chief Complaint

The first major section of an H&P, Chief Complaint, is a very concise answer to the question "Why is the patient seeking medical care today?" It may be a few words or at most a few sentences. Chief Complaint section is sometimes called Presenting Problem or Presenting Complaint. When stated using the patient's own words, it should be enclosed in quotes. Even if it's only a partial phrase, place a period at the end.

Here are a couple examples:

> CHIEF COMPLAINT
>
> "I feel dizzy."
>
> PRESENTING PROBLEM
>
> Status post motor vehicle accident.

History of Present Illness

The next section, History of Present Illness (HPI), fleshes out the chief complaint by discussing the patient's problem in detail. The dictator also may title this section History of Presenting Problem, History, or HPI.

The HPI is written in narrative format. It typically begins with a brief description of the patient (for example, "a 61-year-old Caucasian female") and then discusses symptoms and events leading up to and surrounding the chief complaint. The information may come from the patient, the patient's relatives, and/or previous medical records. If the patient has received prior treatment or diagnoses related to the chief complaint, those will be described here as well.

Here's an example:

> HISTORY OF PRESENT ILLNESS
>
> This 82-year-old African-American female patient has had progressive weakness, which was worse yesterday and prompted her to go to the emergency room. She was found to have an abnormal chest X-ray and admitted for community-acquired pneumonia. She did have cough and audible wheezing but no chest pain or shortness of breath.

If a heading is dictated in an abbreviated or acronym form, you should expand it unless the facility has explicit rules stating otherwise. Thus, HPI, when dictated as a heading, becomes History of Present Illness.

Review of Past History

The Review of Past History section describes previous illnesses, operations, injuries, and treatments not necessarily related to the present illness. It also reviews family medical history and the patient's lifestyle, all factors that can play into the patient's current state of health. Frequently, this information is collected through a questionnaire the patient completes in the waiting room, which is subsequently reviewed with the healthcare provider. If one of the history subject areas has no relevant information, it often will be mentioned anyway to document that it was reviewed.

Depending on the dictator and facility preferences, the review of past history may be grouped into one paragraph under the single heading Past History or broken out into individual major headings. The paragraph format looks like this (and the individual headings are covered in the following sections):

PAST HISTORY

The patient had a CVA involving the right side with left-sided weakness about 15 years ago and has completely recovered. Since then, she has been active and walks daily. No past surgeries. Family history noncontributory.

Past Medical History

Past Medical History (PMH) is limited to illnesses, injuries, and treatments received in the past, except surgical procedures, which are placed under a separate heading. It may be a narrative description or simply a list of conditions. If the conditions are numbered, list them vertically and place a period at the end of each item.

PAST MEDICAL HISTORY

Remarkable for hypertension and seasonal allergies. She has been recently diagnosed with asthma. Vaginal birth x2.

Past Surgical History

This section covers operations and procedures the patient has previously received. They may be dictated in narrative format, as in the Past Medical History example (see the preceding section) or as a numbered list. When numbered, list the items vertically and place a period at the end of each item:

PAST SURGICAL HISTORY

1. Appendectomy at age 12.

2. Hernia repair in 2008.

Family History

The Family History is a rundown of medical conditions experienced by close relatives, which often means the patient is at increased risk of experiencing them as well.

FAMILY HISTORY

Mother with history of coronary artery disease. Brother with history of depression and "nervous breakdown."

Note that "nervous breakdown" is in quotes to indicate that it's an expression of the history-provider's own words and isn't a formal medical diagnosis. In situations like this, the dictator will usually dictate something similar to: "quote nervous breakdown unquote."

Social History

The Social History section includes information about occupation, marital status, living arrangements, and activities. Alcohol use, smoking, or illicit drug use may be included in this section or broken out under a separate Habits heading.

Here's an example:

SOCIAL HISTORY

The patient is a retired plumber. He takes care of his wife, who suffers from Alzheimer disease. Nonsmoker. Drinks very occasionally.

Allergies

The Allergies heading is always included in an H&P. Any allergies are typed in capital letters to make them stand out. Allergies to Medication may be dictated as an alternate heading. If NKDA, an acronym for "no known drug allergies," is dictated, it should be spelled out.

ALLERGIES: No known drug allergies.

ALLERGIES: ALLERGIC TO CODEINE AND DEMEROL.

Current Medications

This section details medications and over-the-counter supplements the patient currently takes. It includes vitamins and herbal supplements, as well as prescribed drugs. In a hospital H&P, this is often referred to as Medications on Admission. This section may be dictated as a numbered list or strung together in a paragraph. Dosage information may or may not be included; it's often left out on admission because the patient may not know it.

MEDICATIONS ON ADMISSION: Aspirin, Procardia, and multivitamins.

CURRENT MEDICATIONS

1. Celexa 20 mg p.o. in the morning for depression.

2. Ativan 0.5 mg for anxiety every 6 hours as needed.

3. Vitamin D daily, dosage unknown.

Review of Systems

The Review of Systems (ROS) is a systematic inventory of potential symptoms the patient may be experiencing, organized by body system. Alternative headings include Systemic Review and Functional Inventory. It also may be referred to as a 12-Point Review of Systems. As with the Past History, much or all of this section may originate from a form the patient fills out in the waiting room.

The ROS may be dictated in paragraph form with no headings or divided into subtopics. Although the subtopic ordering generally starts with the patient's head and proceeds downward, the exact division and arrangement won't always be the same. If there is no meaningful information for a particular body system or even the entire inventory, the dictator may say "noncontributory" or something similar or even skip this section entirely. The use of well-known abbreviations in subtopic headings is permissible and common.

Here's an ROS organized by subtopic:

REVIEW OF SYSTEMS

CONSTITUTIONAL: No history of fever, rigors, or chills.

ENT: No blurred vision or double vision. No headache.

CV: As above.

RESPIRATORY: No shortness of breath, PND, or orthopnea.

GI: No abdominal pain, hematemesis, or melena.

NEURO: Negative.

Here's an ROS in paragraph form:

REVIEW OF SYSTEMS: The patient does not complain of any headache, vision changes, hearing changes, constitutional symptoms, shortness of breath, chest pain, bowel or bladder disturbances, joint or muscle aches, or depression or anxiety symptoms.

REVIEW OF SYSTEMS: Otherwise negative except as in HPI.

Physical Examination

The Physical Examination (PE) is an objective assessment of the patient's condition. The examiner observes, pokes, and prods the patient and records the results here. In some report types, a brief, focused exam may be conducted, but an exam done as part of an H&P typically assesses the patient from head to toe, one body system at a time. Although a PE can be dictated as a narrative paragraph, in an H&P it's more common for each body area to be listed individually, resulting in an outline like this:

PHYSICAL EXAMINATION

General: (The patient's overall appearance.)

Vital signs:

HEENT: (An acronym for head, eyes, ears, nose, and throat; usually grouped together but may also be broken out as individual subheadings.)

Neck:

Lungs (or Respiratory or Chest or Pulmonary):

Heart (or Cardiovascular):

Back:

Abdomen:

Genitourinary:

Rectal: (Frequently omitted or "deferred" for obvious reasons.)

Extremities:

Musculoskeletal:

Skin:

Neurologic:

Psychiatric: (Frequently omitted as extraneous.)

The preceding example shows mixed-case subheadings, but some facilities use all uppercase subheadings instead.

Additional headings that can appear in a full PE, though less common are: Integumentary (skin, hair, and nails), Lymphatic, Genitalia, Breasts, and Pelvic.

The General subheading relays observations about the patient's appearance and demeanor. It usually starts with the patient's age, race, gender, and physical appearance and may include details about emotional state. A typical example:

General: This is a 32-year-old well-developed, slightly obese Hispanic female in no acute distress, alert and oriented x3.

If this information was already provided earlier in the report, the general subsection often is omitted. The rest of the Physical Exam subheadings are self-explanatory.

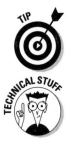

Appendix B provides examples demonstrating how to transcribe phrases commonly dictated in the PE section of a report.

The Review of Systems and Physical Examination may appear to cover the same ground, but they provide entirely different perspectives of a patient's condition. The Review of Systems is a subjective (patient-provided) view of the patient's condition. It's influenced by memory, what the patient is willing to disclose, variations in individual sensitivity to pain, and other personal factors. The Physical Examination gives an objective (examiner-provided) view of the patient's condition as determined by physical evaluation and thus isn't skewed by the patient's feelings, opinion, memory, or mood.

Diagnostic Studies

Diagnostic Studies includes laboratory test results and findings from imaging studies such as X-rays, CAT scans, and MRIs. EKGs and EEGs are reported in this section, too. Instead of lumping these together under Diagnostic Studies, dictators may break them into separate headings, such as Laboratory Data and Imaging.

Conversely, a dictator may dictate the heading Laboratory Data instead of Diagnostic Studies and then include findings from MRIs, EKGs, and other diagnostic procedures, which are technically not lab results. In this case, the MT may modify the headings for clarity, typically by inserting an additional heading immediately below the Laboratory Data section.

LABORATORY DATA

White count 9, hemoglobin 14.8, platelet count 322. Sodium 131, potassium 4.3, chloride 101. BUN 14, creatinine 1.3.

IMAGING STUDIES

Head CT is currently pending. Chest x-ray unremarkable.

Assessment and Plan

Alternative titles for this section include Impression, Diagnosis, and Conclusion. Because an H&P is conducted at the time of a new patient encounter, there often isn't enough data to reach a firm diagnosis yet; the patient's condition is still being assessed and test results may be pending. Therefore, this section often lists provisional diagnoses or itemizes symptoms and conditions that clearly exist and need to be further investigated rather than final diagnoses. Sometimes the assessment and plan will be dictated as distinct sections, each with its own heading.

It's pretty rare for a patient to have a single condition, so items in this section are typically listed vertically as a numbered list. If there's only one item, don't number it, even if the dictator does. Place a period at the end of each item listed, even if it's only one word or a partial phrase.

All abbreviations or acronyms dictated under this heading should be expanded, even if previously defined in the report, unless

✔ The abbreviation has more than one possible expansion and you're not crystal clear on which one it refers to.

✔ It refers to a disease entity that's better known and recognized by the abbreviation than the expanded name, such as AIDS or HIV.

✔ It refers to a non-disease entity such as a lab test (for example, BUN), unit of measure (for example, cm), or medical device (for example, BiPAP mask).

An assessment and plan dictated as a unit looks like this:

ASSESSMENT AND PLAN

1. Chest pain. Cardiac enzymes are negative x2. We will continue aspirin and statin. We will obtain adenosine Myoview stress test today. If negative, okay to discharge to home.

2. Hypertension. Blood pressure is stable. Continue diuretic.

3. History of gastroesophageal reflux disease (GERD). Continue omeprazole.

When dictated separately, the format will be similar to this:

ASSESSMENT

1. Urinary dysuria.

2. Left flank pain

PLAN

Rocephin 1g IM was given. She is to call her primary care physician tomorrow morning in case a second dose is needed. If not, she will fill a prescription for Omnicef 300 mg capsule 1 p.o. b.i.d. for 10 days.

If a patient is referred to a consultant or specialty clinic, or for hospitalization, the new healthcare provider often will perform a separate H&P, which revisits the patient's story from a particular angle. For example, an obstetrician's version of an H&P will place greater emphasis on findings and symptoms associated with pregnancy and childbirth and may provide only a cursory review of the cardiorespiratory system.

Body parts: H&P verbal shortcuts

Running through a list of body systems is a repetitive and often time-consuming process. To speed up things up, dictators make liberal use of acronyms and other verbal shortcuts. Here are some shortcuts commonly used to identify body systems in the Review of Systems or Physical Examination sections of an H&P:

✔ **Cor:** Heart

✔ **CR:** Cardiorespiratory

✔ **CV:** Cardiovascular

✔ **ENT:** Ears, nose, and throat

✔ **GI:** Gastrointestinal

✔ **GU:** Genitourinary

✔ **GYN:** Gynecologic

✔ **HEENT:** Head, eyes, ears, nose, and throat

✔ **NP:** Neuropsychiatric

Chapter 11

Consultation

· ·

In This Chapter

▶ Styling a Consultation report in block or letter format

▶ Surveying the report sections

· ·

A Consultation report is used to convey findings and opinions of a healthcare provider other than the patient's primary physician. It's one of the "Big Four" reports that comprise the heart of most medical transcription work. The consultant assesses the patient's current condition and needs and then suggests or confirms a treatment plan.

Consultations are especially frequent in hospitals, where an emergency room (ER) physician makes an initial assessment and then calls in relevant specialists. It may be to request an assessment of the need for surgical intervention, a cardiology assessment, a psychiatric evaluation, or advice on managing kidney failure.

Primary care physicians often call on specialists as well. A patient with an eye condition may visit his family practitioner, who then refers him to an ophthalmologist, who in turn requests a consultation with a retinal specialist. The patient may visit the consultant just once or return multiple times for treatment and follow-up. Each visit generates a report to the primary care provider and for the patient's chart.

Consultation reports vary in length from a few paragraphs to several pages, depending on the complexity of the case.

In this chapter, I cover all the sections of a Consultation report that you're likely to find. But first I start with an overview.

For more on formatting reports, turn to Chapter 6.

A sample full Consultation report is included in Appendix C.

Overview

A consultation may be dictated as a formal report (called *block style*), organized into sections with headings, or it may be dictated as a letter to the referring physician. Although it isn't an unbreakable rule, dictation for an in-hospital consult is likely to use the formal block format. The letter style is more common for reports on consultations performed during an outpatient office visit.

Consultation reports cover many of the same content areas as a full History and Physical Examination report (see Chapter 10), though the sections are shorter go into less detail. A Consultation report may contain some or all of the following sections:

✔ Identification of referring and consulting physicians and consultation date

✔ Reason for consultation

✔ History of the condition necessitating the consultation

✔ Details of the patient's medical history, including previous medical conditions and surgeries, social and family history, medications, and allergies

✔ Review of symptoms currently reported by the patient

✔ Physical examination findings, frequently limited to the body part or system being assessed

✔ Laboratory data and results of diagnostic studies

✔ The consultant's conclusion regarding the patient's diagnoses

✔ Recommended treatment

Individual consultation reports will vary in exactly which report sections are included.

Consulting and Primary Physicians

Consultation reports begin by specifying the patient's demographic information, date of consultation, and the names of the referring and consulting physicians. Occasionally, additional physicians involved in the patient's care will be listed here as well. Depending on the dictation platform in use, the demographic information may be prefilled for you, or you may be able to select it from a list using the patient's name and date of birth or patient ID number as stated by the dictator when beginning the dictation. The result will look similar to this:

PATIENT NAME: Roper, Skip

PATIENT MR#: 306754

DATE OF CONSULTATION: 00/00/0000

PRIMARY CARE PHYSICIAN: Francis Brindamour, MD

CONSULTING PHYSICIAN: Adam Baum, MD

CARDIOLOGIST: Nick O'Tyme, MD, FACC

If any information is pre-filled for you based on information entered by the dictator, keep in mind that dictators occasionally make mistakes when entering the patient and physician IDs into these systems. You should always verify that the information matches what the care provider dictates.

Reason for Consultation

The headings Reason for Consultation and Chief Complaint are used interchangeably to answer the question "Why is the patient here?" This will be just a few words or, at most, a few sentences. The text may be transcribed on the same line as the heading or beneath it, according to facility preference. Even if it's a partial sentence, place a period at the end. The following two examples demonstrate how this would appear in a block style report:

REASON FOR CONSULTATION

I was asked by Dr. Brindamour to see the patient for chest discomfort.

CHIEF COMPLAINT: Chest discomfort.

If the Consultation report is being dictated as a letter to the referring physician, the reason for consultation will be presented in the opening paragraph, often immediately following a "thank you" to the referring physician.

Dear Dr. Brindamour,

I had the pleasure of seeing your patient, Stanley Cupp, today MM/DD/YYYY in consultation. The patient was referred for evaluation of chest pain.

Details of Present Illness

Immediately following the brief statement identifying the reason for the consultation, the dictator will give a detailed description of the patient's current problem. This may be dictated under the heading History of Present Illness,

History of Presenting Illness, History, or another variation thereof. This is essentially a recap of what was reported in the patient's initial History and Physical Examination report, plus any additional information the consultant obtained from the patient.

HISTORY OF PRESENTING PROBLEM

This is a 61-year-old gentleman with known coronary artery disease, status post 2-vessel stenting in 2009. He presented complaining of several days of not feeling well and feeling lightheaded upon standing. He had noticed some mild and constant chest discomfort and came to the ER and was subsequently admitted for cardiology workup. He recently had his ARB medication changed from one to another.

If dictating a letter, the physician will skip the heading and continue dictating the information as part of the opening paragraph, like this:

As you are aware, Mr. Cupp is a 61-year-old gentleman with known coronary disease status post 2-vessel stenting in 2009. . . .

Review of Past History

Next, the dictator reviews details of the patient's medical and personal history. This can run from a few sentences in a letter to multiple sections in a block-style report. It will incorporate one or more of the following sections:

- ✓ **Past medical history:** Summary of ongoing and previous medical conditions and past surgeries in a list or paragraph format.
- ✓ **Allergies:** Whether the patient has any known medication allergies.
- ✓ **Medications:** A list of current medications and dosages.
- ✓ **Social history:** Whether the patient smokes, drinks, or uses illicit drugs. This sometimes includes information about marital status and current living situation.
- ✓ **Family history:** Medical conditions experienced by family members.

Consultation report elements can overlap the initial H&P to such a degree that some dictators will bypass some or all of these elements and say "Please refer to the patient's chart for history of the present illness, past medical history, allergies, and medications." Typically, you type that verbatim, but in facilities that enable the transcriptionist to access previous patient reports, you may be expected to open the admitting H&P and copy the information into the Consultation report. Your client or employer will tell you which to do.

The dictator may include only sections that have direct bearing on the current illness:

FAMILY HISTORY

Father died of a heart attack at the age of 69. No other pertinent history.

In letter format:

Family history is positive for a father who died of a heart attack at age 69. No other pertinent family history.

Chapter 10, which details the History and Physical Examination report format, goes into greater depth on the type of information potentially included in the preceding sections.

Current Symptoms

The dictator will next describe any current symptoms the patient is experiencing:

REVIEW OF SYSTEMS

All systems reviewed were negative.

Here's the letter format:

Review of systems was negative.

Laboratory and Diagnostic Findings

If there are any pertinent laboratory results or diagnostic studies, they'll be dictated just before or immediately following the physical examination.

DIAGNOSTIC STUDIES

EKG: Normal sinus rhythm, no ST changes. Chest x-ray: Clear with no evidence of heart failure.

Letter version of the same information:

His EKG was reviewed. It shows normal sinus rhythm with no ST changes. Chest x-ray was clear with no evidence of heart failure.

Physical Examination

The physical exam dictated in a Consultation report typically focuses on the body parts and systems closely related to the condition for which consultation is sought. Depending on the type and severity of the patient's condition and physician preference, it can be a full-blow physical examination, but a brief exam covering only the relevant systems is more common.

PHYSICAL EXAMINATION

Temperature is 97. Blood pressure is 125/67. After standing, blood pressure was 110/68. Heart rate did not change and was in the 60s. Respiratory rate is 14. The patient is alert, awake, in no distress. Head and eye examination normal. Jugular venous pressure was 7 cm. Lungs were clear to auscultation. Cardiac exam shows normal S1, S2. Extremities are warm with mild edema. Distal pulses are 2+ and equal.

A consultation letter presents the same information, usually in a new paragraph with no heading:

On examination today, his temperature is 97. Blood pressure is 125/67. After standing. . . .

Impression and Recommendations

Following the history and review of data, the consulting physician provides an assessment of the patient's condition and recommends a plan of treatment. In a formal report, these sections will resemble the following:

IMPRESSION

1. Atypical chest pain, likely noncardiac in nature.

2. Hypertension with orthostasis after a change in medication.

3. Mild lower extremity edema, likely secondary to venous insufficiency.

RECOMMENDATIONS

1. Discontinue the angiotensin receptor blocker (ARB) given the orthostasis.

2. Outpatient pharmacological stress test, which has been scheduled for him.

A Consultation letter takes a less formal approach but conveys the same information:

> I believe the patient's chest pain is noncardiac in nature and due to the change in his ARB medication. His mild lower extremity edema is likely secondary to venous insufficiency.
>
> At this time, I would recommend stopping his ARB given the orthostasis. His other medications should continue as currently prescribed. He has not had a stress test recently, and I have scheduled him for an outpatient pharmacological stress test.
>
> Thank you for asking me to see this patient in consultation.

Chapter 12

Operative Reports

*O*perative reports are the most complex dictations you'll transcribe. The third member of the "Big Four," operative reports give a blow-by-blow account of a surgical procedure. Any time one human being cuts open another and starts tinkering with her insides, it's important to record precisely what was done, down to the last detail.

Certain operations are more common than others, and you'll come to know them very well. By the time you've transcribed your sixth appendectomy, you'll know the steps in such detail that it'll seem possible you could perform one yourself. If you're ever stranded on a desert island and a companion develops appendicitis, just whip out your Swiss Army knife (hopefully, it's sharp) and perform an appendectomy on the spot, saving his life. From then on, he'll have to collect all the firewood and do the dishes, too.

In this chapter, I cover all the sections of an Operative report that you're likely to find. But first I start with an overview.

For more on formatting reports, turn to Chapter 6.

A sample full Operative report is included in Appendix C. Appendix B demonstrates transcription of commonly dictated phrases, including suturing and bandaging examples.

Overview

Operations aren't just performed in hospitals; they're also done in outpatient surgical centers and specialty clinics. An operative report is dictated immediately afterward, detailing who did what to whom using what materials and methods. A full operative report will include the following:

- Preoperative and postoperative diagnoses
- Names of physicians and assistants involved in the procedure
- Title of the procedure performed
- Type of anesthesia used
- Reason the procedure was performed
- Operative findings
- A step-by-step narrative description of the procedure, including instruments used, specimens or tissues removed, any hardware or devices inserted, and wound closure and bandaging details
- Any complications or unexpected developments encountered
- The patient's condition at the end of the procedure and where he was taken afterward

Operative reports cover all these topics, but the level of detail varies substantially based on the complexity of the procedure. Some Operative reports break out each topic with a specific heading; others consist of pre- and postoperative diagnoses, procedure name, and one long narrative encompassing everything else. You should transcribe the report exactly as dictated. Don't insert additional headings or otherwise attempt to organize the report for clarity.

The majority of the examples in this chapter comply with heading and layout styles recommended in *The Book of Style for Medical Transcription*, 3rd Edition, by AHDI. A few stray from the BOS to demonstrate other common layouts you're likely to encounter, such as a heading and data appearing on the same line rather than on separate lines. When transcribing, you should always format reports and headings as specified by the account you're working on, regardless of what standards may otherwise apply.

If a surgeon performs a particular operation frequently, she'll often dictate large portions of it virtually identically every time. You can take advantage of this by creating shortcuts for those parts in your word expander software. When the dictator starts a known section, you can whip out entire paragraphs with a few keystrokes. A word or phrase may change here or there, so be sure to adjust what you auto-inserted to exactly match the current report. Chapter 9 discusses word expanders in detail.

Physicians and Assistants

The first section of an operative report states the date of the operation and spells out who should get credit (or blame) for the results. Many modern transcription platforms fill in the surgeon's name automatically. Surgical assistants, and occasionally the anesthesiologist, also may be named here, and you'll likely need to add those manually.

The current standard is to omit periods between letters in professional designations such as MD and PA, but some facilities still prefer they be included. Most lines in medical reports end in a period, but names are an exception. The result should look similar to this:

SURGEON

Ivana Kutzov, MD

FIRST ASSISTANT

Pansy Ford, PA-C

ANESTHESIOLOGIST

Gibbon Gass, MD

Preoperative and Postoperative Diagnoses

The pre- and postoperative diagnoses immediately follow the names of the surgical team members. If there's a single diagnosis, don't number it. List multiple diagnoses vertically as a numbered list. End each line with a period. Remember to expand any abbreviations or acronyms in the diagnoses section into their full form to comply with the general formatting guidelines described in Chapter 6.

PREOPERATIVE DIAGNOSIS

Menorrhagia.

POSTOPERATIVE DIAGNOSES

1. Menorrhagia.

2. Uterine fibroids.

3. Pelvic adhesions.

If the pre- and postoperative diagnoses are identical, the dictator may lump them together as "pre- and postoperative diagnoses." You should still transcribe them as distinct sections. The quickest method is to copy the preoperative diagnoses list and insert it immediately following the first list. Change the second heading to Postoperative Diagnoses and you're done.

In the preceding paragraph, note that *pre-* has a hyphen after it. When multiple suffixes (in this case *pre-* and *post-*) with the same root appear in a row (often with the word *and* between them), the proper punctuation is to append a hyphen to all but the last suffix. You'll encounter this a lot with *pre-* and *post-*. For additional punctuation help and examples, see Chapter 6 and Appendix B.

Procedure Performed

This section will be titled Procedure Performed, Operation, Operative Procedure, or something similar. If there's a single procedure, don't number it. Otherwise, transcribe the procedures as a vertical numbered list. End each line with a period. This is another report section where abbreviations and acronyms should always be expanded. A procedure list should look like this:

OPERATIVE PROCEDURES

1. Right shoulder arthroscopy with subacromial decompression.

2. Arthroscopic acromioclavicular (AC) joint resection.

If the dictator uses a singular form of a heading, such as *diagnosis* or *operation* but lists multiple items beneath it, transcribe the heading in its plural format, such as *diagnoses* or *operations*.

Anesthesia

This section, usually quite brief, specifies the method of anesthesia used during the procedure. Anesthetics often are used in combination (for example, local with IV sedation). Occasionally, the anesthesiologist also will be named here. This section appears similar to the following:

ANESTHESIA

General endotracheal administered by Dr. Gassor.

ANESTHESIA: MAC.

Table 12-1 lists the types of anesthesia you'll hear dictated most often. Having an idea of which types of anesthesia are used for what can help you decipher difficult-to-understand dictation.

Table 12-1	Commonly Dictated Anesthesia Terms
Type of Anesthesia	*Commonly Used in Surgeries For . . .*
General, general endotracheal	Any surgery where the surgeon wants the patient totally unconscious and unaware
Local	Local numbing for minor procedures
Epidural	Surgical procedures and pain relief from the chest downward, including childbirth and C-sections
Spinal	Surgical procedures below the umbilicus
Interscalene block	Shoulder, upper-arm, forearm
MAC, IV sedation	Colonoscopy, upper endoscopy, and other uncomfortable procedures that don't require general anesthesia
Bier block	Arm below the elbow, leg below the knee

Indications for Procedure

This section, sometimes titled simply Indications, gives a brief summary about why the patient is undergoing the operation. Some dictators include it and others don't. It should be transcribed in paragraph format, like this:

> The patient is a 37-year-old female who injured her right knee while playing hockey approximately 4 months ago. She continued to have pain despite exercise and anti-inflammatories, thus indicating the need for arthroscopy.

Findings

This section gives the surgeon's observations regarding the anatomic structures visible during the operation. Surgical findings may be incorporated into the Description of Procedure section that comes next, but they're often dictated as a separate section instead or in addition, like this:

FINDINGS

Extensive adhesions of omentum and somewhat the colon to the abdominal wall in the right abdomen from his prior open cholecystectomy. The tumor itself was about 4 cm in diameter. It was in the ascending colon just proximal to the hepatic flexure. There was some inflammatory change around it. There was no gross adenopathy. There was no gross evidence of metastatic disease.

FINDINGS: A type II SLAP lesion with instability of the biceps.

Description of Procedure

This section is the meat of an Operative report. Common alternative headings include Procedure in Detail and Operative Technique. It provides a blow-by-blow account of the operative procedure from start to finish. Some Operative reports consist of only preoperative diagnoses, postoperative diagnoses, and this section. The description can run from a half-dozen sentences to multiple pages, depending on the complexity of the operation and individual dictator habits.

The procedure description is transcribed in paragraph format. For short Operative reports, a single paragraph is sufficient. Longer reports are another story. Think about reading an entire newspaper article written as one long paragraph — not much fun! You can greatly improve the readability and, thus, clarity of longer reports by inserting paragraph breaks. Deciding where exactly to insert them is largely subjective, which means you get to decide. Don't stress about this too much — there are multiple legitimate ways to paragraph any long surgical narrative.

If a dictator does specify paragraph breaks, transcribe them as dictated, unless they're blatantly awkward or incorrect. For example, some dictators have a habit of specifying "new paragraph" after every sentence, which results in a very fragmented report. In such cases, use your judgment to create paragraph breaks in appropriate places. Paragraphs should be separated by a blank line.

When some dictators say "new line," they mean new paragraph. You'll be able to determine when that's the case based on context and as you become familiar with personal styles of individual dictators.

If a surgeon dictates a novella-length Procedure in Detail with no paragraph breaks, insert them as appropriate. It's often easiest to type the entire section and then go back and look for paragraph opportunities while proofreading. A new paragraph should be inserted when the topic changes. Logical points include the following:

- ✔ Between a description of preparation and the beginning of the procedure, if the preparation is more than a sentence long.
- ✔ Between the description of the dictator's initial inspection of the relevant anatomy and when she starts to actually do something to it.

✔ In a multipart procedure, insert a paragraph break when the operation proceeds from one stage to another. A good clue is a phrase such as "Attention was then turned to the . . ." or "Next, . . ."

✔ Just before the description of wound closing and bandaging.

Here's a sample surgery description with appropriate paragraph breaks:

DESCRIPTION OF PROCEDURE

The patient was brought to the OR and was given Ancef 1 g intravenous antibiotics. Bier block anesthesia was performed. The limb was then prepped and draped in a sterile fashion.

With that completed, a palmar-based incision was made for an open carpal tunnel release. The transverse carpal ligament was incised with a complete distal and proximal incision. The median nerve was identified and protected at all times. With the procedure complete, irrigation was performed.

A simple closure was performed with 3-0 nylon, and a bulky Bunnell-type dressing was applied. The tourniquet was deflated. The sponge, needle, and instrument counts were found to be correct. The patient was awakened and taken to the recovery room in stable condition.

Disposition

The Disposition section records where the patient went after leaving the operating room. Sometimes it also includes instructions or plans for the immediate postoperative period.

DISPOSITON: The patient was transported to the recovery room in stable condition.

DISPOSITION

The patient will be discharged to home with instructions to elevate the extremity; maintain the dressing clean, dry, and intact; and follow up in the office in 72 hours for a wound check.

Additional Headings

The previous headings are the ones most commonly included in an Operative report. The sections may be dictated in a different order or use alternative heading wording. Depending on the type of operation performed and dictator and facility preference, a report may include additional headings.

Complications

This heading is used to call attention to any complications or unexpected circumstances encountered during the surgery. Often this information is included in the Details of Procedure section, but it may also be given its own heading. It's almost always as follows:

COMPLICATIONS

None.

Tourniquet time

A tourniquet is sometimes used during a procedure to prevent blood flow to the area being operated on. In such cases, the amount of time the tourniquet was in place is usually specified.

TOURNIQUET TIME

16 minutes.

Estimated blood loss

This heading specifies how much bleeding occurred during the procedure. Usually it simply says "minimal," but occasionally it's more specific.

ESTIMATED BLOOD LOSS

Minimal.

ESTIMATED BLOOD LOSS: Less than 5 mL

Drains

At the conclusion of surgery, a tube may be placed to permit fluids to drain from a wound. When this is done, it will be mentioned in the procedure details or under a separate heading, like this:

DRAINS

One 1/8-inch Hemovac drain.

Hardware and implants

Operations that involve inserting something into the patient's body and leaving it there will detail exactly what that something was. A pacemaker may be placed or an intraocular lens inserted. Orthopedic operations frequently involve placement of enough screws and miscellaneous parts to stock a small hardware store. Items such as these are described in detail in the Operative report, either within the procedure description or under a separate heading, as in the following:

HARDWARE

Biomet mini-balance femoral stem, size 10; a Biomet metal-on-metal acetabular shell, size 58; with a 52 standard-size femoral head.

IMPLANT

Alcon Laboratories model MC50BD, 25.0 diopter lens.

Specimens

When body tissue is removed from a patient, it's often sent for pathological examination. It may be an entire organ, such as a patient's gallbladder, or some other tissue such as a tumor or cyst. The removed tissue is called a *specimen,* and it will be listed in the operative report, like this:

SPECIMENS

Bilateral palatine tonsils.

SPECIMEN: Appendix sent to Pathology

Sewing Up the Case

Nearly every surgery wraps up with wound closure. Similar to a seamstress sewing a quilt, a surgeon sewing up a person has a large variety of stitches and threads from which to choose. When a dictator describes how she sutured something, she may mention suture size, suture material, and the suturing method, usually in that order.

Suture sizes range from 11-0 (smallest) to 7 (largest). Dictators pronounce the zero as "oh," so "one oh nylon sutures" should be transcribed as 1-0 nylon sutures. If the dictator says "number one oh nylon sutures," place a # sign where the dictator says "number":

Dictated: number one oh nylon sutures

Transcribed: #1-0 nylon sutures

The 0 in a number-0 combination refers to a quantity of zeros in a row. Thus, #4-0 sutures means size #0000 sutures, which are a much smaller than #4 sutures. Dictating or transcribing 0000 is cumbersome and error-prone, so the format 4-0 is used instead.

The type of suture material usually follows right after the size. It may be stated as a trade/brand name, such as "Prolene" or using a generic term, such as "polypropylene." There are many, many types of suture material. Here are the ones you'll encounter most often:

absorbable	Ethibond	silk	Dacron
fast-absorbable	Ethicon	Vicryl	Tevdek
Prolene (polypropylene)	Ethilon	Mersiline (polyester)	PDS
	chromic		steel
nylon	catgut	Monocryl	Nurolon

Next up is the manner in which the sutures are deployed, frequently dictated as "in a *something* fashion" or "using *something* technique." Here are words commonly used in this section:

simple	subcuticular	tension	Halsted
interrupted	subcutaneous	retention	Lembert
running	locking or interlocking	figure-of-eight	
horizontal or vertical mattress	over-and-over	purse-string	

Often several of them will be strung together, as in:

using interrupted vertical mattress technique

When a dictator says "oh vicryl" it means 0 (zero) Vicryl.

Dictators, being dictators, may alter the order or omit the suture size, material, or suturing method, but if you're familiar with the structure, it's usually easy to understand what they're saying.

Chapter 13

Discharge and Death Summaries

· ·

In This Chapter

▶ Examining the sections in a discharge report

▶ Detailing diagnoses, operations, and medications

▶ Recapping treatment history and hospital course

▶ Transcribing a death summary

· ·

Discharge summaries are the final member of the "Big Four" family of medical transcription reports. They're among the most interesting to transcribe, because unlike other members of the core four, they don't leave you hanging, wondering how things turned out for the patient. A History and Physical Examination (H&P) report tells you how the story starts but then puts you on hold. Operative reports and Consultation reports provide glimpses of what happens in the middle. A Discharge Summary wraps everything up into a nice, neat package. A Death Summary, of course, records the details of a patient's final discharge.

Example Discharge Summary and Death Summary reports are included in Appendix C.

Discharge Summary

Each time a patient is released from a hospital, rehabilitation facility, or other in-patient care setting, a Discharge Summary is generated. The patient may be going home, transferring to another facility, or sometimes just moving to another department in the same facility. The Discharge Summary serves as a sort of patient hand-off document for whoever sees the patient next.

Overview

A Discharge Summary provides an overview of a patient's hospitalization from admission through discharge. It can be a few brief paragraphs or a multipage report, depending on the complexity of the patient's condition and treatment. A typical report covers the following topics:

- Admission and discharge dates
- Names of physicians involved in the patient's care
- Initial and final diagnoses
- Key laboratory and diagnostic data
- A list of operations and medical procedures performed
- A chronological narrative of the patient's progress from admission through discharge
- Medications the patient is on at the time of discharge
- The patient's condition when discharged
- Post-discharge instructions and plans

The layout, format, and sections included in a Discharge Summary vary between facilities and sometimes even among dictators at the same facility. The majority of the examples in this chapter comply with heading and layout styles recommended in *The Book of Style for Medical Transcription*, 3rd Edition, by AHDI. A few stray from *The Book of Style* to demonstrate other common layouts you're likely to encounter, such as a heading and data appearing on the same line rather than on separate lines. When transcribing, you should always format reports and headings as specified by the account you're working on, regardless of what standards might otherwise apply.

The first thing a Discharge Summary does after stating the admission and discharge dates is name names. The patient's primary care provider gets top billing, followed by specialists involved in the patient's care. Some transcription platforms will insert the names automatically, but others will require you to type some or all of it in. If it's already present, confirm that it matches what's dictated, because a finger slip somewhere along the way can result in a wrong patient or physician ID being entered into the system. A typical Discharge Summary heading will start out like this:

PATIENT NAME: Newman, Anita

ADMITTED: 00/00/0000

DISCHARGED: 00/00/0000

PRIMARY CARE PHYSICIAN: Kerry Oakey, MD

NUTRITIONAL CONSULTANT: Holden D'Mayo, MD

A dictator may supply a department name instead of a person's name:

CONSULTANTS: Nephrology and Hematology.

Admitting and Discharge Diagnoses

A Discharge Summary may include both Admission and Discharge Diagnoses or just Discharge Diagnoses. They're typically dictated in list form, usually near the beginning of the report. They should be formatted as a numbered list unless the facility specifies otherwise. If a diagnosis is dictated using an abbreviation or acronym, it should be expanded to its full form and followed by the acronym in parentheses. So, "DVT" becomes "deep venous thrombosis (DVT)."

If the admitting and discharge diagnoses are identical, and the dictator may give them in one fell swoop as Admission and Discharge Diagnoses. You should transcribe them as separate lists anyway. The quick and easy way is to copy the admitting diagnoses list and change the title of the copy to Discharge Diagnoses.

Typical Admitting and Discharge Diagnoses lists look similar to this:

ADMISSION DIAGNOSES

1. Cerebrovascular accident (CVA) with left arm weakness.

2. Hyperlipidemia.

DISCHARGE DIAGNOSES

1. Cerebrovascular accident (CVA) with left arm weakness and MRI indicating subacute infarct involving the right posterior parietal lobe.

2. Hyperlipidemia.

Don't be thrown for a loop if a dictator dictates primary and secondary diagnoses instead of admission and discharge diagnoses. When a patient has multiple coexisting conditions, the heading Primary Diagnosis is sometimes used to highlight the patient's immediate problem; everything else is stashed under the heading Secondary Diagnoses.

If the dictator says "Admitting Diagnosis" but lists multiple conditions, change the section title to the plural format, Admitting Diagnoses.

History

The History section, also dictated as History of Present Illness or Brief History, provides introductory information about the patient and the circumstances leading up to admission to the facility. It's often essentially a reiteration of the same section from the patient's admitting History and Physical Examination (H&P) report, although perhaps worded differently. Given the degree of overlap, dictators sometimes just reference the H&P instead of repeating it.

BRIEF HISTORY

A 3-year-old boy with a history of asthma. On the night of admission he complained he was having trouble breathing, and his mother brought him to the ER. He was noted to have subcostal retractions, expiratory wheezes, and O2 saturation of 97% on room air. He was given albuterol nebulizer treatment and subsequently admitted to the pediatric floor.

HISTORY OF PRESENT ILLNESS

Please refer to admitting History and Physical Examination for full details of history and presentation.

Hospital Course

The Hospital Course describes the patient's progress and treatment between admission and discharge, in chronological order.

HOSPITAL COURSE

The patient underwent L5-S1 Gill decompressive laminectomy and posterior lumbar interbody fusion with pedicle screws with general anesthesia. She tolerated the procedure well. She did complain of some persisting numbness in the S1 dermatome of the right foot postoperatively. She was ambulatory, and her pain was under control with oral analgesics at the time of her discharge.

A patient's History of Present Illness and Hospital Course are frequently combined under History and Hospital Course, Hospital Course, or Course in Hospital.

Laboratory Data

The Laboratory Data section of a Discharge Summary includes only values directly relevant to the patient's diagnosis and treatment, not every test that was administered. A dictator may emphasize this point by titling this section Pertinent Laboratory Data.

Diagnostic studies such as an MRI, CAT scan, and EKG often are dictated along with the lab results. However, if facility specifications permit it, it's good practice to break them out into a separate section with an appropriate heading, like this:

LABORATORY DATA ON ADMISSION

BMP unremarkable. White blood cell count 8.1, hemoglobin 12.0, hematocrit 36.2, platelets 180,000. Urinalysis negative. Culture negative.

IMAGING

Principal imaging while in the hospital included CT of the head, which showed no evidence of acute intracranial hemorrhage.

Procedures Performed

This section lists major procedures or operations performed during the patient's hospitalization. It doesn't include routine items such as starting an IV, only "big stuff" like an operation, insertion of a feeding tube, or another special procedure. Principal Procedures Performed and Operations Performed are common alternative titles for this section.

When there's only one procedure, it will look like one of these (depending on how the facility prefers section headings to be formatted):

OPERATION PERFORMED

Right total knee replacement.

PROCEDURE PERFORMED: Right total knee replacement.

If there are multiple procedures, they should be listed vertically and numbered. As with other numbered lists, end each line with a period. If a procedure name is dictated using an acronym or abbreviation, expand it to its full form. For example, "LV angiogram" would become "left ventricular (LV) angiogram."

A list of multiple procedures should look like this:

PROCEDURES PERFORMED

1. Left heart catheterization.

2. Coronary arteriogram.

3. Left ventricular (LV) angiogram.

4. Successful percutaneous transluminal coronary angioplasty (PTCA) of the mid left anterior descending (LAD) stenosis, reducing it to about 20% to 30%.

Physical Examination on Discharge

Most discharge summaries include a discharge physical examination. It usually pales in comparison to the formality and scope of an admitting physical, but it often includes similar headings. A discharge exam may be limited to the body systems immediately relevant to the patient's diagnoses. Frequently, the discharge exam is expressed in paragraph format, even if the admitting exam is customarily transcribed in a vertical format at the same facility. When in doubt, check previous reports from the facility to confirm the preferred layout.

PHYSICAL EXAMINATION

At the time of discharge vital signs were stable. HEENT: Pupils equal and reactive to light. Extraocular movements normal. Neck: No JVD or bruits. CVS: S1, S2 normal. Lungs: Clear to auscultation bilaterally. Abdomen is soft, nontender, nondistended, with positive bowel sounds. Extremities: No pedal edema. Neurologic: Nonfocal. Skin: No rash. Surgical incision looks clean.

Turn to Chapter 10 for the head-to-toe details about what's included in a full physical examination.

Discharge Medications

Every discharge summary includes a list of medications the patient is taking at the time of discharge. It includes medications the patient was already taking on admission and incorporates modifications or additions. The items should be formatted as a numbered list with a period at the end of each line.

1. Vitamin C 500 mg daily.

2. Symbicort 2 puffs twice a day.

3. Duragesic patch 25 mcg per hour q.72 h.

Some facilities use a system called medication reconciliation to track a patient's medications. All medication orders from admission through discharge, including any dosage adjustments, are recorded on a single form. Dictators at facilities that use this system may dictate the following instead of a list:

DISCHARGE MEDICATIONS: See medication reconciliation list.

Plan/Disposition

The final section of a Discharge Summary records the patient's medical status at the time of discharge and whether he's going home or somewhere else. If any follow-up appointments have been arranged, they may be listed here as well. The topics may be broken out into separate headings or dictated as a single paragraph, depending on the dictator's habits and preference. When dictated as individual sections, it will appear similar to this:

CONDITION ON DISCHARGE

Improved.

DISPOSITION

Discharged to home.

ACTIVITY

As tolerated.

When dictated under a single heading, it will resemble this instead:

PLAN

His condition at the time of discharge is stable. Activity as tolerated. Diet is a cardiac diet. Follow up with primary care physician.

Discharge Instructions

Dictators may break out instructions given to the patient or a caretaker at the time of discharge as a separate heading.

DISCHARGE INSTRUCTIONS

Maintain splint, clean, dry, and intact. Utilize ice to the left ankle as needed. Follow up with Dr. Finklefifer on Monday at 8:30 a.m.

Additional headings

The previous sections are the most common, although they may be dictated in a different order or use alternative wording for the headings. There are a few more you'll encounter from time to time. Reason for Admission or Reason for Visit may be given near the top, immediately before the History section. It states the reason for the patient's admission in the briefest possible form:

REASON FOR ADMISSION: Renal colic.

An allergies heading may be included, but usually only if the patient has any:

ALLERGIES TO MEDICATION: CODEINE.

Occasionally, especially if the patient is leaving the hospital in less than ideal shape, a Prognosis heading is added.

PROGNOSIS: Poor.

Some Discharge Summaries conclude with a sentence specifying the amount of time the physician spent preparing the patient's discharge. This is used to determine billing codes, and you should include it in the transcription even though it often sounds more like a comment than part of the official report.

Time spent: More than 45 minutes.

Death Summary

When a patient dies, the Discharge Summary becomes a Death Summary. Transcribing a Death Summary can be somewhat heart wrenching, especially when it's clearly sudden and unexpected or involves a child. Often the dictator's tone of voice will reveal feelings of regret, although in other cases the doctor is very matter of fact about it. Fortunately, Death Summaries are one of the least common report types.

A Death Summary contains a subset of the normal Discharge Summary headings. Key differences include the following:

✔ Discharge Date will be replaced by Date Expired or Date of Death.

✔ Discharge Diagnoses will be replaced by Final Diagnoses.

✔ Cause of Death may be dictated as an explicit heading.

It's common for a death summary to contain only Final Diagnoses and Hospital Course sections. Occasionally, the dictator will give a narrative description with no headings at all.

If you encounter a death summary that particularly upsets you, don't hesitate to e-mail or call a fellow MT. You can't reveal patient specifics due to privacy concerns, but you can give a general description of the circumstances. Often just sharing the information will help you feel better.

Chapter 14

Beyond the Big Four: Other Common Reports

● ●

In This Chapter

▶ Noting proceeding details

▶ Charting progress with soap notes

▶ Delivering the details of childbirth

▶ Recording radiology results

▶ Gathering official opinions

● ●

*T*he History and Physical (H&P) report, Consultation report, Operative report, and Discharge and Death summaries are the stars of medical transcription work, but they're supported by a staff of additional reports. This chapter introduces some of the more prominent staff members, what their jobs are, and how to handle them.

The majority of the examples in this chapter adhere to the heading and layout styles recommended in *The Book of Style for Medical Transcription,* 3rd Edition, by AHDI (see Chapter 6). A few of the examples stray from the BOS to demonstrate other common layouts you're likely to encounter, such as a heading and data appearing on the same line rather than on separate lines.

When transcribing, you should always format reports and headings as specified by the account you're working on, regardless of what standards may otherwise apply.

Procedure Notes

Procedures range from placement of a feeding tube, to cardioversion to correct a heart rhythm, to a colonoscopy — pretty much anything that doesn't require a full-blown operating room (OR) and surgical team. Many procedures are diagnostic in nature, such as electroencephalographies (EEGs), sleep studies, and cardiac stress tests. The reports may detail a procedure done in a physician's office, at a hospital bedside, or in a specialty clinic. Some simply name the procedure and then give a brief summary of the process and pertinent findings; others are precisely formatted and include procedure-specific subheadings. The first thing all of them do is identify the procedure, like this:

PROCEDURE PERFORMED

Colonoscopy.

Indications for Procedure

The body of a procedure note begins by explaining why the procedure is being performed:

INDICATIONS FOR PROCEDURE

This is a 72-year-old female with a history of rectal bleeding.

Alternative section names include Preoperative Diagnosis and Reason for Procedure, or sometimes, when more detail is included, History.

Medications

When a list of the patient's current medication is dictated in a procedure note, the medications should be numbered and listed vertically.

CURRENT MEDICATIONS

1. Ambien.

2. Plavix.

Unlike a patient's full medication list, anesthesia or procedure-related medications don't need to be numbered or formatted vertically unless the facility specifies it.

PREMEDICATIONS

Versed 5 mg, Demerol 75 mg IV.

Procedure in Detail

The body of the report provides a narrative description of the procedure. This section is also commonly given the title Technique.

PROCEDURE IN DETAIL

The Olympus video colonoscope was introduced into the rectum and advanced under direct visualization to the cecum and into the terminal ileum. No abnormalities were seen of the terminal ileum, the ileocecal valve, cecum, ascending colon, hepatic flexure, transverse colon, splenic flexure, descending colon, rectosigmoid, and rectum. Retroflexion exam in the rectum revealed no abnormality. The colonoscope was withdrawn. The patient tolerated the procedure well.

If a procedure includes measurements as part of the procedure process, they often will be interwoven into the narrative. To see this in action, check out the *polysomnography* (a fancy word for sleep study) in Appendix C.

Findings and Recommendations

When not already stated at the beginning of the report as postoperative diagnoses or bundled into the procedure description, the results of a diagnostic study appear in a section titled Findings, Conclusion, or Impression, similar to this:

FINDINGS

1. Small internal hemorrhoids.

2. Otherwise unremarkable colonoscopy.

RECOMMENDATIONS

High-fiber diet. Repeat colonoscopy in 5 years.

Chart and Progress Notes

A chart note, also called a progress note or office note, is dictated when an established patient is seen for a repeat visit. A chart note records the reason for the current visit, an assessment of the patient's condition (including any changes since the previous visit), and additional treatment rendered or planned. A chart note may be as short as a few lines, especially for a follow-up visit. A new problem may warrant several paragraphs.

Because chart notes are often so short, some offices will have you transcribe multiple notes into a single document. They'll be split apart later after the physician has reviewed them. They can be dictated in a variety of formats, including

- Like a mini H&P, with similar headings but less depth
- As a single paragraph (often just a few sentences)
- Using SOAP note format or a close variation (most common)

SOAP is an acronym for:

Subjective: The reason the patient is being seen, including description of symptoms provided by the patient or other individuals.

Objective: Details drawn from the provider's examination of the patient's condition, including lab data.

Assessment: What the provider thinks is wrong with the patient, based on subjective and objective details.

Plan: What the provider recommends be done regarding the patient's condition. This may include obtaining lab work, referral to a specialist, or ongoing treatment and follow-up details.

Given their love of shortcuts and acronyms, it should come as no surprise that some dictators just say the letters S, O, A, and P instead of the full headings.

Some dictators use a different set of abbreviations to accomplish the same thing:

CC: An acronym for chief complaint, equivalent to subjective

PX or PE: Shorthand for physical examination, equivalent to objective

DX: Abbreviation for diagnosis, equivalent to assessment

RX: Abbreviation for prescription, in this case prescribed treatment plan

A dictator may omit sections or mix and match headings. For example, he may dictate Chief Complaint in place of or in addition to Subjective but otherwise follow the SOAP acronym. He may inject additional headings, such as Lab Data or ROS (Review of Systems) along the way. You should transcribe whichever headings are dictated unless you've been specifically instructed otherwise.

In addition to the patient's reason for seeking care, the subjective heading often incorporates background data, creating a mini history, like this:

SUBJECTIVE: He is here for evaluation of back pain. He has had persistent back pain which was somewhat improved by PT but has been severe and disabling. He cannot walk or bend over very well, but he is slowly improving. He is taking Flexeril and Vicodin.

In fitting with the condensed nature of chart notes, most facilities format chart notes with the text starting on the same line as the heading. It's also common to indent the text from the heading, like this:

> S: A 90-year-old here for a follow-up on her medical issues, which include atrial fibrillation and valvular heart disease.

The Objective section may be just a sentence or two about the relevant body part, like this:

> OBJECTIVE: She does have some swelling around the anterior ankle.

Or reference another document:

> OBJECTIVE: See labs.

It may be replete with jargon, abbreviations, and acronyms to jam a physical exam into as small a space as possible, which you should transcribe as dictated:

> O: Lungs clear. Cor nl. S1, S2, neg. S3, S4, murmur. Abdomen neg. h/s meg., masses, tenderness. Ext's no edema.

In a dictation like the preceding one, the only way you're going to have a fighting chance of understanding the dictator is to refer to her previous reports.

The Assessment and Plan sections may be separate or combined. There's no need to number multiple diagnoses unless the dictator does. Nor do you need to expand diagnoses acronyms in SOAP notes, even though you would in most other report types:

> A: DM type 2. Depression, improved.
> P: Reviewed glucometer usage. Reviewed his diet.

A combined Assessment/Plan section would resemble this:

> A/P: Atrial fibrillation: Stable. Good rate control. Continue anticoagulation at this time.
> Pneumonia: Improving on Zithromax day 3/5.

Appendix C demonstrates chart and progress notes in several formats.

Radiology and Imaging Reports

Plain X-rays, MRIs, CT scans, and ultrasounds are just a few of the multitude of techniques used to diagnose and treat our diseases and injuries. They offer the power to visualize and reach parts of the body without resorting to surgery for a direct inspection — a definite plus for the patient!

Imaging studies often involve a *contrast medium,* or dye, either taken orally by the patient or injected. The distribution of the dye highlights particular anatomic features, making them easier to identify and examine.

Imaging technologies also are used during surgery to guide the movement of surgical instruments or deliver a treatment to a particular body part without creating any substantial holes to get there. For example, if a patient has a suspected heart attack, an interventional radiologist can insert a catheter via a small incision in the patient's leg, direct it through the arterial system to the heart, and use it to identify and remedy any blockages, using imaging to direct every step.

Radiology and imaging reports record

- The type of imaging study performed and body part being studied
- The quantity and type of views recorded
- Contrast materials or medications used
- The reason for the study
- A description of the test process, if relevant
- The results of the study
- Conclusions and recommendations

A study can have multiple parts. Often initial images will be recorded; then some change will be made, such as manipulating the patient's limb, having him run on a treadmill, or administering contrast dye or medication; and then repeat images will be taken.

Imaging studies are sometimes dictated as operative reports or procedure notes, particularly if the procedure was performed in an operating room, as may be the case with a procedure that involves anesthesia or accessing a region deep inside the body, such as the spine or heart.

Study details

The initial section of a radiology report relays the specifics of the study. It describes the types of images obtained, contrast material or medications used, and any relevant circumstances/comments, such as bowel preparation protocol for a colonoscopy.

> PROCEDURE: MRI, left knee, without contrast.

If the results are being compared to results of a previous study, the date and name of the comparison study will be given here or under a Comparison heading.

Reason for Study

This section briefly states the reason for the study. Alternative titles include History, Clinical History, or Indication. This tends to be a few words or a few sentences at most, like this:

> REASON FOR STUDY: Chest pain.
>
> CLINICAL HISTORY
>
> The patient is a 70-year-old man with worsening lower back pain and bilateral lower extremity weakness.

Technique

This section describes how the procedure was performed, along with the nature of the images obtained. For something straight-forward, like a plain X-ray, it will be as simple as:

> TECHNIQUE: PA and lateral views were obtained.

A complex procedure, such as cardiac angiography, may include a step-by-step narrative that runs several paragraphs long.

What's a view? Think of an X-ray machine as gun and the film that records the image as a target. Picture yourself standing between the gun and the target while someone pulls the trigger. If you're facing the gun, then the X-rays will pass through your body from front (anterior) to back (posterior) on the way to the target (the film). The resulting image is called an AP (anteroposterior) view. If you turn sideways to the gun, the X-rays will shoot in one side of you and out the other, creating a lateral (from the side) view. If you position yourself at a 45-degree angle to the gun, the X-rays will pass through you at an angle, creating an oblique view. Get the picture?

Findings

The measurements, values, and observations recorded during the study are reported here. This section also may be titled Interpretation or Results. The findings may be presented in a narrative format, a series of subheadings with associated values, or a combination. The format is highly dependent on the type of study and facility preferences. Here's an example of renal ultrasound findings:

FINDINGS

The right and left kidneys measured 4.9 and 5.0 cm in length, both near the lower limit of normal in size. The kidneys are otherwise normal in appearance and normal in position. The bladder is full and normal appearing on transverse images.

Incidentally, there is a low-attenuation mass measuring 1.7 x 1.4 x 1.8 cm within the inferior aspect of the left lobe of the liver.

Occasionally a study uncovers something unrelated to the condition that prompted the investigation, like the liver mass in the example above. These are referred to as incidental findings. Tumors (usually benign) are found by coincidence commonly enough to have an official name: incidentalomas.

Impression

The report concludes with the radiologist's assessment of the significance of the findings. It can be as specific as a list of diagnoses or a more general "is suggestive of" narrative.

Summary of Labor and Delivery

A summary of labor and delivery, or delivery note, is a brief recap of events that occur immediately before and during childbirth. If the mother undergoes a C-section, a separate operative note is dictated. A delivery note may be dictated with preoperative (pregnant) and postoperative (delivered) diagnoses or as a descriptive narrative with no subheadings. In either case, it describes

- ✔ The mother's condition on arrival, including stage of labor and results of prenatal lab tests

- ✔ Any interventions, such as anesthesia, an episiotomy, or the use of Pitocin to augment labor or forceps or suction to aid delivery

✔ The mother's condition after delivery

✔ The infant's time of birth, delivery position, gender, weight and length, and condition at birth

Special terminology is used to summarize the mother's obstetric history. There are two systems used for this: GPA and TPAL. GPA is an acronym for gravida (number of pregnancies), para (number of live births), and abortus (miscarriages or induced abortions). The A (sometimes referred to as Ab) is frequently dropped if zero. Thus,

A 23-year-old G2, P1 white female

describes a woman in her second pregnancy, with the first one resulting in a live birth. A dictator may use the actual terms instead of the letters; in either case, separate them with commas.

TPAL is an acronym for term births (T), premature births (P), abortions (A), and living children (L). TPAL numbers should be separated by hyphens. If a dictator gives a series of four numbers as the obstetric history, it should be transcribed like this:

A 23-year-old 2-2-0-2 white female

A dictator may mix and match GPA and TPAL systems. You should transcribe it however she dictates it. See Appendix B for helpful examples.

Another term specific to delivery notes is Apgar score. Apgar is an eponym (Dr. Virginia Apgar invented the test) that's also used as an acronym. The acronym, which shouldn't be expanded, stands for appearance, pulse, grimace, activity, and respiration — a checklist used to quickly assess a newborn's condition on a scale of zero to ten. Every delivery note mentions at least two Apgar scores, one from one minute after birth and one at five minutes, like this:

A viable female infant with Apgar scores of 7 and 9.

An example summary of labor and delivery is included in Appendix C.

Psychiatric Assessment

A full psychiatric evaluation is performed when someone is admitted to a hospital or outpatient mental health program and again on discharge. They're also frequently prepared by psychiatrists and psychologists when taking on a new patient. The examiner asks a lot of personal questions and weaves the answers into a comprehensive report that is drawn on to develop a treatment plan and referred to on future visits.

A psychiatric assessment is likely to land in your job queue in the form of a consultation report or discharge summary. A report that incorporates input from family members and others in the patient's social circle (often referred to as informants) can go on for pages. When the only information source is an uncooperative or incapable patient, you'll have a lot less to transcribe. Topics commonly covered include

- ✔ Reason for current admission/referral
- ✔ Previous psychiatric history
- ✔ Substance abuse concerns
- ✔ Family and personal social history
- ✔ Medical status, including any physical ailments and current medications
- ✔ Current mental status, as assessed by the examiner
- ✔ Psychiatric diagnoses or possible diagnoses

Much of the information in a psychiatric evaluation is obtained by questioning the patient or through the examiner's observations. When practical, family members and significant others may be interviewed as well.

A psychiatric report occasionally includes a physical examination, but often that is left to a separate H&P report. The exception is when the patient's current psychiatric condition may be related to a physical injury, such as a blow to the head. In a situation like that, a full physical exam may be included or at least referred to.

Presenting Problem

The first thing a psych report does is address the question: Why is the patient here today? It's not unusual for the practitioner and the patient to provide different answers! If the answer contains words stated verbatim from the patient or another informant, they should be placed in quotes.

In a consultation report, the heading is typically Reason for Referral. In a hospital or clinic, it may be History of Present Illness or Reason for Consultation. Chief Complaint is also an option.

REASON FOR CONSULTATION

Dr. X, the patient's primary care provider, referred her to me for evaluation and treatment of anxiety.

PRESENTING PROBLEM

"I'm so stressed out that I dread getting up in the morning."

The presenting problem in a hospital report is likely to be more dramatic:

HISTORY OF PRESENT ILLNESS

The patient is a 42-year-old female who was found wandering around the mall parking lot and appeared intoxicated. According to police, she kept asking shoppers to help her "get the chickens out of my pockets." She was brought to the ER by EMS.

CHIEF COMPLAINT

"Why am I here?"

The presenting problem, or case introduction, is often much longer than these examples.

Past Psychiatric History

This section reviews any previous mental health treatment or diagnoses the patient has received. This, again, can be quite long:

PAST PSYCHIATRIC HISTORY

The patient was first hospitalized at 14 years of age. This is his 5th hospitalization. The first one occurred when. . . .

Or extremely brief:

PAST PYCHIATRIC HISTORY: Denied.

Substance Abuse

This section relays details of the patient's substance use or abuse, as self-reported and per past medical records. The title may vary, but the meaning is clear:

ALCOHOL AND DRUGS

The patient admits to marijuana use in the past but not currently, denies alcohol or tobacco. No history of treatment for alcohol or drug problems.

SUBSTANCE ABUSE: Denies.

Past Medical History

Any significant or ongoing medical conditions or surgeries are listed here. There's no need to number them unless the dictator does.

PAST MEDICAL HISTORY

Medical history is notable for factor V Leiden deficiency, restless leg syndrome, and migraine headaches.

Family History

Mental health issues of immediate relatives, such as parents, siblings, and children, are described here. This tends to stick to mental health history: things like suicide, schizophrenia, alcoholism, or Alzheimer's. If potentially relevant family medical issues exist, they're often placed under a separate heading.

FAMILY PSYCHIATRIC HISTORY

Her mother has depression. Her son has ADHD. No known family history of suicidal attempts or completions. No history of drug or alcohol issues in the family.

FAMILY MEDICAL HISTORY

Her mother has migraines. There is diabetes on both sides of the family.

Social History

Pretty much anything is fair game in this section. It typically starts out with demographic information about the patient's circumstances of birth and then progresses chronologically to the patient's current living situation. Relationships, children, deaths, relocation, and traumatic occurrences are described. The patient's level of educational and work history often are mentioned. If the patient has legal issues, such as a child custody dispute or criminal charges or convictions, they may be listed here as well.

All this is frequently wrapped into a single narrative and transcribed in paragraph format. If the narrative is long, you may insert appropriate paragraph breaks for clarity, but don't reorganize or otherwise neaten it up, even if it's long and rambling. A dictator may use subheadings to divide the social history into sections. Common alternative titles for this section include Psychosocial History and Social and Developmental History.

SOCIAL HISTORY

The patient is single, never married. He has a 4-year-old daughter living in Texas, which he admits makes him sad. He is a high school graduate. He works at an automobile dealership as a service manager. He says his job is very stressful and he is constantly worried about losing it. He is estranged from his family of origin and has little social support. No current unresolved legal problems.

Current Medications

If the patient regularly takes medications, they'll be listed here. This section may be dictated as a numbered list or strung together in a paragraph. If the dictator numbers them, list the medications vertically with a period at the end of each line.

CURRENT MEDICATIONS

1. Lexapro 10 mg per day.

2. Valtrex 500 mg per day.

Mental Status Examination

The mental status examination (MSE) assesses the patient's current mental state. It describes the patient's appearance, attitude, behavior, mood, thought process, and other aspects of her current condition.

Dictators tend to stick to favorite phrases, making them good candidates for entry into your word expander (see Chapter 9).

MENTAL STATUS EXAM

Adult female appears stated age, cooperative, noted to have some scars on her right forearm, disheveled, not in any acute distress or anxiety. Speech is appropriate, able to engage adequately in conversation, denies any auditory or visual hallucination, denies any suicidal or homicidal ideation, thoughts, plans, or gestures. Mood: She reports as depressed. Affect: Constricted. Insight and judgment are poor.

Despite very similar names, a mental status examination (MSE) and mini-mental state examination (MMSE) are different tests. The MMSE assesses cognitive function by testing memory, ability to do simple math, and whether the patient knows where she is and what time it is. The MMSE is often used as a screening test for dementia. An MMSE is only occasionally dictated as part of a psych evaluation.

Diagnoses

Psychiatric diagnoses are expressed using a format that is distinct from all other medical diagnoses lists. They are organized into a five-part structure called a multi-axial system. Each axis covers a different aspect of the patient's condition and can include multiple items. The axis number is expressed using Roman numerals. The dictator will state the axis number and the diagnoses associated with it, resulting in a structure like this:

DIAGNOSES

Axis I

1. Schizoaffective disorder, bipolar type.

2. Rule out depression.

Axis II

Deferred.

Axis III

Upper respiratory infection.

Axis IV

Financial pressures.

Axis V

GAF is 50.

The axis number and heading may be written on the same line or on separate lines, per facility preference. When on the same line, the text should be separated from the subheading by a tab, in a format similar to this:

PROVISIONAL DIAGNOSES

Axis I:	Mood disorder, NOS; generalized anxiety disorder.
Axis II:	Deferred.
Axis III:	Hypothyroidism. History of low vitamin D.
Axis IV:	Good social support.
Axis V:	Current GAF 25.

Psychiatric diagnoses use very specific wording that comes from the _Diagnostic and Statistical Manual of Mental Disorders_ (DSM) published by the American Psychiatric Association. The DSM has been around since 1952, and a dictator may specify the edition he's using. Editions are identified by appending the version number using Roman numerals. Extra letters may be tacked on the end, such as *R* for revised edition or *TR* for text revision, as in the following examples:

DSM-III-R DSM-IV DSM-IV-TR

The acronyms GAF and NOS are frequently used in psychiatric diagnoses. Global Assessment of Functioning (GAF) is a numeric score (0–100) used to subjectively rate a patient's social, occupational, and psychological level of functioning. NOS is an acronym for "not otherwise specified" and is often deployed as a synonym for "I'm not sure." Its use indicates that a patient's problems fall into a particular family of disorders (for example, anxiety disorders or depressive disorders), but there's not enough information available to categorize it further.

Treatment Plan

The final section lays out the next steps for the patient, such as hospital admission, medication changes, or follow-up appointments.

> TREATMENT PLAN: She will be admitted to the inpatient psychiatric unit under the care of Dr. Jones and placed on suicide precautions. Her current medications will be continued for now.

Independent Medical Evaluation

An independent medical evaluation (IME) is a comprehensive review of a patient's medical history performed by a physician not previously involved in the patient's care. IMEs are usually performed for a legal purpose, such as assessing eligibility for workers' compensation or disability benefits or for litigation related to an accident or injury. A qualified medical evaluation (QME) is the same thing as an IME. Topics covered in an IME include:

✔ Factors surrounding the onset of the patient's illness or injury

✔ A detailed description of the patient's medical course and treatment, including a full review of available records

✔ Consideration of any additional information, such as a report provided by a private investigator

✔ A physical examination

✔ Assessment of the appropriateness of the care already rendered

> ✔ Whether further medical care is warranted
>
> ✔ Determination as to whether the patient has a permanent disability and its exact nature and degree

Although any physician can complete an IME, there are companies that specialize in providing them. The requestor contacts the IME provider, which then taps into its network of specialists to find a qualified evaluator. The majority of IME work comes through companies such as these, and they can be a good source of interesting transcription work.

Standard medical transcription formatting guidelines are largely ignored in favor of customized formatting that fits on letterhead stationery. Section headings, for example, may be centered, transcribed in mixed case instead of uppercase, bolded, underlined, or any combination thereof. The formatting and organization of IME reports is also more diverse than any other report type. It's essential to obtain a model report or template to use as a starting point, even though the sections dictated may vary.

An example IME is included in Appendix C.

Introduction

The first thing an IME does is state the name of the patient, the date of the injury or onset of illness, and the purpose of the report. If the report is related to an insurance or disability claim, a case number is given.

> Re: Patient, Unfortunate
>
> DOB: 02/13/1977
>
> Case #: 23159777
>
> Date of Injury: 11/01/2011
>
> Date of Examination: 11/25/2012

The first paragraph summarizes the purpose of the report:

> As requested by Verribig Insurance Company, I evaluated Mr. Amos Stake in my office on November 25, 2012, for injuries sustained to his left hand on November 1, 2011, during the course of his employment as a forklift operator at Widget Manufacturing Co. The purpose of this review is to address the issue of long-term disability related to his hand injury.

History and Present Complaints

The history of the case may be given in a single large section titled History or be divided into subheadings. In either case, it's usually very extensive. It provides details about who the patient is and how he came to be in his current condition. If the injury is employment related, it will include a work history going back for years.

Many of the subheadings used in the history portion of an H&P also are used here, including past medical and surgical history, social habits, and family history. Each encounter with a medical provider may be listed by date and described. When compensation is being sought for a disability, a great deal of attention will be focused on the patient's physical and mental capabilities before and after the incident. Almost anything can be pulled in; if the report requestor hired a private investigator to follow the patient around and watch for signs of malingering, perhaps going on a ski vacation while allegedly too injured to work, that will be mentioned here as well.

Transcribe exactly as dictated. If you have the slightest doubt about a word or phrase, flag it for dictator review.

Physical Findings

Occasionally an IME is based purely on review of records, but more often there's an in-person examination as well. The exam often is limited to body parts/systems related to the reason for the IME but can go into those in fine detail, resulting in something like this:

> Hand grip strength, as measured by Jamar dynamometer, showed left hand at 49, 44, and 51 pounds; right hand at 50, 57, and 45 pounds. Lateral pinch gauge using Jamar pinch gauge showed left hand at 17.1, 17.2, and 16.2 pounds; right hand at 16.2, 16.3, and 17.5 pounds. Circumferential measurements of both upper extremities showed left arm at 25.2 cm, left forearm 21.3 cm; right arm 24.4 cm and right forearm 21.4 cm.

Diagnostic Studies

The examiner will review and comment on the results of laboratory tests, MRIs, and other diagnostic studies. The discussion may be under this heading or incorporated into another section.

Records Review

An IME often includes an itemized list of documents that the examiner reviewed as part of the evaluation. These reports are from office visits, treatments, and diagnostic procedures the patient received. The records list may be dictated near the beginning of the report as part of the introduction, or just before the examiner renders his conclusions. It should be formatted as a vertical numbered list, like this:

Medical Records Review:

1. January 22, 2011: Annual physical exam by the patient's primary care. No patient complaints reported.

2. March 15, 2011: First report of injury. X-rays of the left knee were negative.

3. April 12, 2011: MRI of the left knee showed complete tear of the mid to distal ACL.

Diagnosis

The diagnosis section of an IME can stray quite far from other medical documents. Of particular note, diagnoses should be transcribed exactly as dictated without expansion. Diagnoses are usually formatted as a vertical list. So, the diagnoses section of an IME may look like this:

Diagnoses:

It is my opinion that the diagnoses are:

1. Mild residual left shoulder weakness with full range of motion.

2. Residual pain in left medial epicondyle area.

3. Left wrist weakness.

An IME report doesn't always include a separate diagnosis section. The diagnosis may not be in dispute, or it may be discussed in the introduction or conclusion of the report rather than listed under a distinct heading.

Conclusion

This is where IME reports get wildly divergent. Their purpose is to either answer a question or give a determination regarding degree of disability and prognosis. The resulting conclusion sections commonly take one of three formats:

✔ A simple yes/no opinion and rationale

✔ A series of answers to specific questions

✔ A set of headings related to rating degree of disability

Some dictators will employ a combination of conclusion styles.

Yes/No opinions

If the IME has been requested in order to evaluate the need for or appropriateness of a specific treatment, for example a particular operation, then the conclusion is usually a paragraph or two answering yes or no and rationale behind the answer, similar to this (but longer, of course):

> CONCLUSION
>
> It is my professional opinion within a reasonable degree of medical certainty that Mr. Quewl has significant right shoulder adhesive capsulitis consistent with a postsurgical "frozen shoulder." It is my opinion that a repeat arthroscopy for lysis of adhesions is indicated.

Here's another example:

> ASSESSMENT
>
> My opinion is that she is recovered from these injuries at this time. Her treatment appears to have been appropriate. My opinion is she has reached a medical endpoint for the injuries suffered on 1/20/12 and needs no further treatment.

Question-and-answer format

It's very common for the requestor of an IME to ask the evaluator to answer very specific questions, especially if the requestor is an insurance company or attorney. In such cases, the questions and answers to them are listed in the conclusion section of the report, like this:

> **Answers to Specific Questions:**
>
> 1. **Are the current symptoms causally related to the injury that occurred on 11/30/2012?**
>
>   In my opinion, the symptoms are related to the injury of 11/30/2012. The impact of the object onto Mrs. Kersaway's foot. . . .
>
> 2. **Based on your overall clinical assessment and review of records, has the claimant reached maximum medical improvement with regard to the injuries?**
>
>   It is my opinion that Mrs. Kersaway has reached maximum medical improvement and no further treatment is necessary.

Disability assessment headings

The conclusion portion of an IME related to a workers' compensation claim is often structured by headings to determination of disability. Typical headings include:

- ✔ **Disability status:** Is the patient disabled? Permanently or temporarily?

- ✔ **Impairment rating:** Exactly how much permanent impairment has the patient sustained from the injury. This is drawn from a handbook and is very specific, like this:

    Based on the *AMA Guidelines,* 6th Edition, Chapter 16, Mr. Beaderday is entitled to a permanent disability rating of 12% of the lower extremity, which is comparable to 5% whole person.

- ✔ **Causal relationship and apportionment:** Was the injury caused or aggravated by the reported workplace event? If partially, to what degree?

- ✔ **Work restrictions or limitations:** Can the individual continue working? The answer may be with restrictions, not at all, or perhaps in a new profession with vocational training.

- ✔ **Maximum medical improvement (MMI):** Has the patient reached a stable condition that is unlikely to improve further?

Physician Certification

A report that is being specifically created for legal use often concludes with a physician certification. This is often a few sentences describing the examiner's credentials, followed by a place for the examiner to date and sign the report and attest to its accuracy. This may be added to the document after transcription or as part of the transcription process.

Part IV

Employment Matters: Landing and Managing a Medical Transcriptionist Job

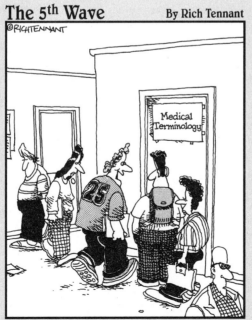

The 5th Wave — By Rich Tennant

@RICHTENNANT

"I'm really pumped to learn some advanced medical terms. I can feel the watchamacallit really flowing through those little round tube thingies in my body."

In this part . . .

This section delivers behind-the-scenes how-to's to help you build your new career. Here, you get tips and advice on how to locate and land a medical transcriptionist job — and then manage the job instead of allowing it to manage you. You also get an assist with the technical details of outfitting a home office, bone up on financial matters of particular importance to freelancers, and discover principles behind working healthy so you can thrive in your medical transcriptionist career for a long time to come.

Chapter 15

Medical Transcriptionist Job Hunting

A really annoying phrase is included in more online MT job listings than not: "At least X years of experience required." The value of X ranges from one to seven, with two being most common. What do you do if you don't have any experience at all yet? First, stop looking at those job boards. There are much better places to start an MT job search, especially if you're a new graduate.

If you've trained appropriately, landing your first MT job isn't nearly as daunting as those job listings may lead you to believe. In this chapter, you find the best places to hunt for MT jobs and get tips to help you along the way. Naturally, one of your first tasks will be to create or polish up your résumé. However, all the polishing in the world won't make work experience magically appear on it. The good news is that a temporary blank spot won't prevent you from getting a job, if you can do well on a pre-employment test. As long as you did well in MT school, passing these tests is mostly a matter of knowing what to expect and applying the strategies in this chapter to give yourself a leg up.

No matter how eager you are to get started, grabbing the first job offer that comes along without fully evaluating it first is a mistake. It may be the perfect position for you, or it may be a nightmare waiting to happen. The information in this chapter helps you know what to look for and which questions to ask, so that you can properly scope things out.

Getting Organized: Prelaunch Planning

It can be plenty tempting to skip the planning part of a job hunt, especially if you're a freshly minted MT eager to get cranking or an experienced veteran whose current employer has gotten on her last nerve. As with so many things in life, however, the more pressure you feel to act immediately, the more you'll gain from pausing to take inventory and get organized before you move forward. Be thoughtful and methodical now so you can be happy with the job you end up in later. Besides, it really only takes minimal time and effort to actually do it!

Identifying your perfect job

Step one is to explore the characteristics your ideal job would have. You have to know what you're looking for so you can decide the best places to look. If you could have any MT job in the world, would it be

- ✔ Full time or part time?
- ✔ As an employee or independent contractor (IC)?
- ✔ Acute care, a particular specialty, or clinic work?
- ✔ Production-based pay or hourly pay?

If you've researched current pay rates and have in mind a minimum starting rate, add it your list. If there are certain hours you absolutely cannot (or are unwilling to) work, specify that, too. These are your starting parameters.

Creating this list doesn't lock you in to anything, and it doesn't mean you should only consider jobs that match it perfectly. It simply provides a ruler you can pull out at any time to measure an option.

Understanding why your first job should be full time

If you're a new MT, consider starting with a full-time position if you can possibly swing it. Even if you ultimately intend to work part-time, starting out full time makes a lot of sense for several reasons:

- ✔ You'll become competent a whole lot faster, which in turn means you'll be able earn more per hour, be frustrated less often, and have more career options sooner.
- ✔ It'll be easier to find a job.

There is a major ramp-up involved in transitioning from excellent student to effective MT. Despite the amazing amount of data you've recently crammed into your noggin, there are many, many more things to master that only come through experience. Hence, that perennial "minimum two years' experience" line. Undertaking a big transition like that on a part-time basis is akin to planning to traverse the Appalachian Trail while only hiking on Tuesdays and Thursdays. At best, it's going to be a long, slow process; at worst, it's never going to happen because you'll end up quitting in frustration. To put it more bluntly, you need to decide whether to quickly rip the Band-Aid off so you can get that part over with faster, or peel it away slowly. Guess which one employers prefer?

Companies who hire just-graduated MTs know all this. Quite understandably, they prefer to hire people who will attain cruising speed and become a contributing member of the team as soon as possible. That doesn't mean you absolutely can't start out part-time, but you'll pay a price for it in multiple ways, including pay rate and ramp-up time.

Once you've got on-the-job cred, you'll find it much easier to drop to working fewer hours and still make a worthwhile income, because you'll be vastly more efficient and effective — and marketable.

Starting with acute care or clinic work

The decision to start with acute care or clinic work is not going to make or break the rest of your MT career, but it does matter. It's a choice better made on purpose than left to chance. To help you decide, here are some characteristics of acute care transcription:

- ✔ You work primarily for hospitals and urgent-care facilities.

- ✔ You work on a large variety of report types crossing numerous specialties and subspecialties, including operations (which many MTs find fascinating).

- ✔ There is a large, often changing pool of dictators, making it harder (if not impossible) to learn their idiosyncrasies and create time-saving shortcuts.

- ✔ There is a heavier concentration of English as a second language (ESL) dictators.

- ✔ You're virtually always required to work at least one weekend day.

- ✔ There is often higher deadline pressure with tighter turnaround times.

- ✔ A greater depth and breadth of skills are needed, which usually translates into a higher rate of pay.

- ✔ Skills are very transferrable to other acute-care or clinic MT positions.

And here are some characteristics of clinic transcription:

- ✔ You work primarily for physician offices and specialty groups.

- ✔ There are fewer report types to master — typically limited to H&Ps, office notes, consultation reports, and referral letters.

✔ There is a smaller pool of dictators, making it easier to learn their idiosyncrasies and create time-saving shortcuts.

✔ The turnaround times are typically not as tight and you're under somewhat less pressure.

✔ You have the potential to earn more money with less stress if the stars align (and you're a master of shortcuts).

✔ The skillset isn't as marketable due to the laws of supply and demand.

✔ The work is more repetitive and potentially less intellectually stimulating than acute care work.

You also can specialize in a field like radiology or oncology, but that's more likely to be an option for experienced MTs than newcomers to the field.

Keeping a log

When you're interacting with multiple potential employers at once, a log file can be a lifesaver (and a face-saver). It doesn't need to be anything fancy, just a place to keep track of your contacts and progress (or lack thereof) with various job prospects. A word-processing document, a spreadsheet, or even a notebook will suffice. Spreadsheets are a particularly flexible option because it's easy to sort the entries by company name, date, status, or any other column you care to create.

As soon as you get a new job lead, add it to your log. Record an initial brief description of the company, the type of work it does, and where you got the lead. Add names and contact details as you obtain them. Going forward, keep notes about your interactions with each potential employer. Include the date, type of interaction (submitted résumé, had a phone interview, took a test, and so on), with whom, and any comments. You don't need to write a book, but record enough so that if they call you out of the blue three weeks from now, you'll know where you left off. Remember to periodically make a backup copy of the entire log, even if simply by printing it out.

Creating a cheat sheet

As you complete applications and interviews, you'll find yourself repeatedly fielding the same questions from different employers. Make it easy on yourself and reuse your answers. Keep them in a text document so you can paste them into an online application form or e-mail and feel confident that they're 100 percent grammatically correct and typo free.

Knowing Where to Find Job Opportunities

Skip the big job boards for now — there are much better places to start your search. The most useful, by far, are

- ✔ The school you obtained your MT training from
- ✔ MTs you know personally
- ✔ MT online communities

This isn't to suggest that MT jobs listed on all-purpose job boards are automatically inferior; however, the vast majority do seek experienced MTs. Speaking of which, if this is your first MT job, you should be seeking an experienced employer — one that has hired new grads before. Getting up to cruising speed on your first MT job will be a lot harder than you anticipate. Even if you breezed through MT school, type blazingly fast, and have a grasp on medical matters that would make Hippocrates proud, it isn't going to be easy. Employers who routinely hire new MTs know what to expect and (hopefully) have processes in place to help you get up to speed.

If you can swing it and the timing works out, a trip to the AHDI Annual Convention and Expo (ACE) is an unbeatable opportunity. Many employers actively recruit there. You also can meet and network with fellow MTs, who may have job leads to share. See when and where the next one is at www. ahdionline.org.

Your training school's job resources

Without question, the first stop on your job hunt should be your MT school. Almost all MT schools have ongoing relationships with potential employers and offer career coaching of some kind. The best will hand you a list of potential employers, complete with contact information and details on the kinds of employment relationships they offer. Even those, however, can't hand you a job — that's something you'll have to earn on your own.

Here are some ways you can leverage your MT school connections:

- ✔ **Ask your training school about job placement assistance they offer, specifically if they have particular employers who regularly hire their graduates.** You probably already investigated that before you enrolled, but it won't hurt to refresh your memory on the details.

✔ **Take advantage of opportunities to network with current and former students.** Most online MT programs include private student message forums. Start frequenting them before you graduate and familiarize yourself with employers that people there are discussing. If there's a graduates-only board, get access to it the minute you're eligible. You may identify employers you definitely don't want to work for, as well as some you'd like to.

✔ **Approach your instructors for advice and recommendations.** They've probably shepherded plenty of students through this process and likely have valuable tips and leads to offer.

Medical transcription websites

Online MT communities should be a key part of your job search for numerous reasons, including the following:

✔ Many of them have job boards or forums where current openings are posted.

✔ They're ideal places to get the scoop on pros and cons about particular employers. You can find out who's hiring, cutting back, merging, and who's treating their employees how.

✔ Medical transcription recruiters hang out in them.

You'll be hard pressed to find a more generous group of people than your fellow MTs. They're avid networkers. Many will freely share their knowledge of particular employers, though you may have to private-message them to get the full scoop. Occasionally, someone will post that his current employer is hiring. Here are a few places you can tune in to MT job listings and employment discussions:

✔ MTDaily (www.mtdaily.com) and its sister site MTJobs (www.mtjobs.com)

✔ The careers section of the AHDI website (www.ahdionline.org)

✔ The Medical Transcription Networking Corner group on Facebook (www.facebook.com/groups/MTCorner)

✔ MTStars (www.mtstars.com)

Take what you read in online forums with a grain of salt. After all, you're only getting one side of the story.

All-purpose job boards

Although they shouldn't be your starting point, general job boards are still worth perusing. Keep in mind that some of the job listings on such boards seem to be semipermanent, perhaps serving more as a way to collect résumés than to fill current job openings. However, if you're looking for a job at an individual facility rather than with a medical transcription service organization (MTSO), these job boards do carry a greater percentage of them. For example, you may uncover an opening at a nearby hospital or medical facility. Two of the better options are Monster (`www.monster.com`) and CareerBuilder.com (`www.careerbuilder.com`).

Crafting Your Résumé

The sharper your résumé is, the better. However, don't pull your hair out over creating a one-of-a-kind, knock-their-socks-off document. Potential employers will primarily be looking for three things:

 ✔ Appropriate training and/or experience.

 ✔ Professional attitude. (You'd be surprised how many new graduates take a casual, inappropriately friendly approach to job hunting.)

 ✔ Attention to tiny details, a highly necessary trait for MTs. That means not one single typo, misspelled word, or grammatical error.

Concise, clear, accurate descriptions paired with traditional fonts and a super-simple layout are highly recommended. Avoid fancy graphic designs, lots of tabbing, and bullet points — they're likely to throw some applicant-tracking technologies for a loop and make the résumé look messy after it's been mangled by the system.

It's a good idea to prepare two versions of your résumé: one nicely formatted and the other in plain text. In some cases, recruiters will ask you to paste your résumé into an e-mail or directly into an online application form instead of submitting it as an attached document. Before submitting it to anyone else, paste your résumé into an e-mail and send it to yourself — you should know what it's likely to look like when it comes out the other end.

Be sure your résumé includes the following sections:

 ✔ **Contact information:** Include your street address, phone number, and an e-mail address that doesn't sound ridiculous. If your phone number changes, be sure to update your résumé with the new one, or you definitely won't get "the call."

✔ **Work history** (how much, when, and what kind). For MT jobs, mention specialties and report types by name. For example:

<u>Magnificent Transcription</u>, Beautiful, NC   Jan 2012–Present

Medical Language Specialist

Transcription of acute care reports for hospitals in Illinois and Maryland, including H&P, discharge summaries, operative reports, consultations, cardiology tests, pulmonary tests. QA score 98%–99%.

✔ **Education, with MT training at the top:** Include school name and graduation date, and describe the curriculum. If you're proud of your GPA, include it; if it's not what you'd hoped for, leave it off, but be prepared to answer questions about it in an interview. Here's a short curriculum summary:

> Trained in advanced medical language, anatomy and physiology, human disease processes, laboratory procedures, technology for the MT, HIPAA laws, formatting and editing using the AHDI *Book of Style.* Extensive hands-on practice with transcribing beginning, intermediate, and advanced dictation, including foreign accents/ESL and using word expanders and productivity software.

✔ **Certifications and memberships:** This is where you list your AHDI student membership and perhaps your RMT credential.

Make sure to incorporate words a recruiter will use when searching a database of candidate résumés. Your résumé may be a beacon of formatting and organizational perfection, but if it doesn't contain the terms recruiters use to search a résumé database, it may vanish into digital oblivion anyway. You probably already have a pretty good feel for trigger words to include. There are a couple easy ways to bolster your starting list:

✔ Read recruiters' minds by reviewing current MT job listings for likely terms.

✔ Search MT résumés on sites such as Indeed (www.indeed.com) to see what your competitors are writing on their résumés.

If you need a little help with formatting and layout, there are lots of books and online articles about crafting résumés, including *Resumes For Dummies,* 6th Edition, by Joyce Lain Kennedy (Wiley). Don't get sucked into the pursuit of a perfect résumé, though; polishing résumés is nice, but time spent prepping for interviews and employment tests matters more.

Facing and Acing Employment Tests

Although it's not unheard of to land an MT job without first taking a pre-employment test, it's very rare. The usual process goes something like this:

1. **You contact the recruiter and submit your résumé.**

2. **The recruiter likes what she sees and gives you instructions for taking and submitting a pre-employment skills test.**

3. **You take the test.**

   The test often has two parts:

   - A medical language/transcription knowledge assessment

   - A hands-on portion in which you complete sample transcriptions

4. **If you do well on the test, the recruiter calls you, conducts a phone interview, and potentially offers you a job.**

   The interview may be with the supervisor of the transcription account you're being considered for rather than the initial recruiter.

It's a good idea to do some advance scouting before submitting an online application. Some MT employers incorporate the test as part of the application submission process rather than in a separate step. In such cases, it starts the moment you hit the Submit button on your application. If you're not expecting it, the surprise factor can throw you off your game.

MT pre-employment tests vary from company to company, but they all have a large psychological component. You're being put on the spot — how will you perform? If you can push test anxiety out of the picture, you'll find them a lot less stressful. Even if you can't completely eliminate test stress, you can drastically reduce it by doing two things:

- Understanding how the tests work and what they're really testing

- Getting some practice so you become familiar with the process

You can knock off the first one by the end of this chapter.

Conquering the mind game

Pre-employment tests are a psychological challenge as much as an intellectual one. Pre-employment tests check up on your technical knowledge, but they also assess additional things, like your ability to follow instructions, deal with technical matters, and make judgment calls.

If you're like many people, when you're put on the spot, you may seize up to some extent and not perform to your true level. A large part of that is simply fear of the unknown. That's why you should never apply to your first-choice employer first. Instead, pick a potential employer farther down on your list. Apply, take its transcription test, interview as appropriate, and repeat. If you're like most new grads, you'll probably fail a pre-employment test or two. Rest assured that the earth will not part beneath your feet and swallow you whole should this occur. Also, keep in mind that if the sample dictations are insanely difficult, it's quite likely the real dictators on the account are, too. If that's the case, ending up with a different employer may not be such a bad thing.

After you have a few rounds under your belt, it's likely your test anxiety will be substantially reduced, and you may even have found your future employer earlier than expected.

Knocking off the knowledge assessment

The knowledge assessment is usually administered first to weed out candidates who don't know *-ectomy* from *-otomy* or can't easily distinguish between words like *their, they're,* and *there.* It consists of multiple choice questions about medical terminology, grammar, capitalization, and punctuation. Occasionally, a few fill-in-the-blank questions will be thrown in. It generally covers very straightforward stuff you'll have no problem with if you've completed a solid MT training program.

Meeting the transcription challenge

The transcription portion typically includes several sample dictations at varying levels of difficulty. At least one of them is likely to be very difficult to understand, possibly to the point where only a seasoned MT with samples from the same dictator to refer to could get it completely right. Because you don't have those, you're really not expected to achieve perfection. Do your best to avoid leaving blanks, but keep in mind that the company may be checking what you'll do when you encounter impossible dictation, so don't be afraid to demonstrate!

Tools to use

Web-based employment tests are usually open book, just like real transcription. Have your references at your fingertips. If you use web-based resources, open them in additional browser tabs before starting the test, so they'll be loaded and ready to go.

When it comes to completing the transcription portion, the two things that matter most are sound quality and how much control you have over the playback process. You'll likely get clearer sound through headphones than through your computer's speakers, so make sure they're plugged in and working.

If you're able to download the sample dictation to your computer and use transcription software to transcribe it instead of playing it via your default web browser settings, you'll almost certainly achieve vastly better sound quality than you would playing it via your default web browser settings. You'll also be able to speed up, slow down, and rewind the transcription files using the transcription foot pedal you used in school, which is much easier than constantly interrupting your transcription to accomplish the same things with the keyboard. If you recently graduated from an MT school, you may be able to do this by using the software and foot pedal you used while training. Many applicants are either unaware of this possibility or are unable to pull it off, so if you can do it, you'll already have an edge over other applicants, and your recruiter will likely be impressed by how much you correctly transcribe in comparison. ***Hint:*** You don't necessarily need to mention how you leveraged technology to do it.

Evaluating and Comparing Job Offers

Resist the temptation to instantly accept the first job offer you receive. At the very least, you need to learn more about the specifics of the job before accepting or declining it. Then give yourself at least a couple days to consider it, especially if your job hunt is young. If you've been at it a while, and this is your first real offer, you'll have to go with your gut on whether to accept it immediately. Even so, ask questions first.

Questions to ask before accepting a job offer

Collecting additional facts before deciding about a job offer is totally routine and acceptable, so don't feel like you're endangering anything by asking.

The list in this section contains recommended questions. Most apply to both IC and employee positions. A few of them, such as questions about mandatory overtime, apply only to employee-status offers.

There are critical differences between working as an IC versus working as an employee. If you're not clear about what those are, be sure to read Chapter 19 before picking one over the other.

Here are some of the questions you'll want to ask:

- ✔ **Is this an employee or independent contractor position?**
- ✔ **What types of accounts and reports will I be transcribing?**
- ✔ **What transcription platform will I be working on?**
- ✔ **Will you provide the necessary equipment, including the computer and software, or do I have to provide it?**
- ✔ **What percent of the dictators is ESL?**
- ✔ **What constitutes a line?**
- ✔ **How do you compensate overtime?**
- ✔ **Are any productivity incentives or shift differentials available?** A *shift differential* means you get paid a little more to work less popular hours. A pay rate has probably already been stated as part of the offer, but if it hasn't, be sure to ask about the pay rate, too.
- ✔ **What happens if I run out of work?** Common answers include the following:
    - You'll have a secondary account you can switch to.
    - You *must* make up the lines later when more work is available.
    - You have the *option* to make it up later if work is available.
- ✔ **Is there ever mandatory over time? If so, how often?**
- ✔ **How long have the accounts I'll be working with been on the speech recognition (SR) system?** (You need to ask this only if your work includes SR editing.) SR system accuracy improves over time and an account that's just been added will be substantially more difficult to work on than one that's been on longer.

It's a good idea to finish with an open-ended question like: Is there anything else I should know? It opens the door to information you haven't specifically asked about.

Delaying acceptance, tactfully

Your goal is to buy a little time to evaluate the offer and perhaps drum up additional offers to compare it to, but without imperiling the one currently on the table. It's a common and reasonable practice, but it can be a little awkward to execute. Having a game plan in mind for this purpose helps.

Here are some tips to help you develop that game plan:

✔ Express appreciation for having received the offer and that you have strong interest in the position.

✔ Explain that you're weighing several offers, emphasizing that you want to be certain you make the right choice for both yourself and your future employer.

✔ Promise to get back with a decision within a specific time frame. A week is pretty standard; going longer than two weeks is probably pushing it.

If you already have another offer on hand or think one is imminent, bring the second employer (Employer B) into play as well. Let Employer B know that you've received an offer from another company and that you've got it on hold because you're really interested in Employer B. Request a decision from Employer B within the specified time frame.

Being mindful of your long-term goals

When you have a specific offer in hand, it's time to pull out the description of your perfect job you created earlier. How does this potential position measure up? You'll also need to conduct some additional research, which can easily be accomplished from the comfort of your keyboard.

Your favorite MT online communities are a great place to start. Search them for recent discussions that mention the potential employer. Ask other MTs you know if they've heard anything good or bad. It can't hurt to type the employer's name into Google and see what pops up.

It's a good idea to research the reputation of the transcription platform as well. Some of them are much better to work on than others. Seven cpl on a platform that boosts productivity and 7 cpl on a platform that hampers it are entirely different propositions.

If you start discussing the employer you just interviewed with on a public MT message board, the recruiter may see it and look upon it unfavorably. Whenever feasible, use private-messaging features and your MT school's forum for such discussions. If a public posting is called for, use tactful phrasing and picture the potential employer standing behind you looking over your shoulder (benevolently, of course) while you type.

Don't be discouraged if your job hunt doesn't produce immediate results. Some MTs, especially those with top GPAs from respected schools, find employment easily. Others have to employ a lot more patience and persistence.

It can be more difficult to land an MT job near the end of the year, because dictation volume tends to drop off over the holiday season. It's something to be aware of, but don't let it prevent you from looking in November and December. It doesn't always hold true, and even when it does, if you impress an employer, they may go ahead and snap you up but delay your starting date until January. Hiring tends to slow down in July and August, too, as doctors, patients, and recruiters head to the beach.

If you're a new graduate and struggling to leave the starting gate, consider deferring your dream job in favor of immediate employment. For example, you may want to

✔ Open yourself to the possibility of working more, less, or different hours

✔ Consider taking an IC instead of an employee position or vice versa

✔ Accept a lower starting line rate than you originally planned on

Sometimes you have to decide whether you're willing to make compromises and do what it takes to get your foot in the door. Then you work your leg in there, and before you know it, you'll be all the way through that first door, and new ones will be opening before you.

If all goes well, you'll be able to land an MT job without ever calling on the foot-in-the-door tactic. Soon after that, the phrase "At least X years of experience required," will become music to your ears, because you'll have it.

Chapter 16

Managing On-the-Job Issues

· ·

· ·

*Y*ou'll probably always remember the day you land your first medical transcription job. After months of challenging training and a job hunt, you finally get to put your skills to work. Leaving the safety of practice dictations for the world of handling real medical records for actual patients is a big step, and it can be a little nerve-wracking. This chapter is here to help ease your transition.

Knowing what's "normal" for a new medical transcriptionist (MT) can go a long way toward relieving rookie anxiety, so that will be the first stop. Next, I explain the process of quality assurance in medical transcription and the role you'll play in it. Protecting patient privacy is another issue you'll deal with on a daily basis. The whys and hows of protecting patient confidentiality surveyed in this chapter will aide you in accomplishing this critical task.

Your First Job: Knowing What to Expect

Before you sit down at your keyboard on that exciting first day of your first MT job, know this: you'll get off to a much slower start than you ever imagined. *This is normal.* The production speed you'll be able achieve when starting your first MT job will most likely be a fraction of what you were hoping for. Rest assured, you'll get much faster — it's just going take longer than you thought it would.

The average full-time MT transcribes somewhere between 1,000 and 1,500 lines per day. It's routine for new MTs to notch 500 lines per day or less — standard, run-of-the-mill, routine. You'll have a lot of things to accomplish, including

✔ Learning the transcription platform

✔ Getting to know the formatting styles and transcription rules of accounts you work on

✔ Starting to build up your expander file and library of sample reports

✔ Becoming familiar with dictator idiosyncrasies

At the same time, you'll face the traditional hurdles of new employment — meeting your supervisor, learning the processes for tracking your work and managing administrative matters, and generally learning the ropes at your new employer.

None of this would be remotely as stressful if you weren't being paid on production, and this is where a little mind game can come in handy: Think of your first month on the job as a continuation of your MT training program. You paid for that training — you're getting *this* training for free! As silly as that may sound, it can take the stress off if you consider this learning time and not earning time.

Most new MTs also do battle with the issue of perfection. They'll go to extremes to avoid those terrible, self-esteem-busting blanks. In fact, that's one of the chief productivity killers: spending tons of time trying to pin down a mystery word rather than leaving a blank. Do the best you can, but cut yourself some slack, too. As a new MT transcribing dictators you've never heard before (some of them probably horribly awful beyond belief), no matter how hard you try, some of your reports are going to have more holes than a block of Swiss cheese. You may actually also format a heading incorrectly or misplace a comma. Horrors!

Fortunately, someone's got your back, and those imperfect reports will never reach a patient's chart. As part of the quality assurance (QA) process, every report you transcribe will automatically be put "on hold" and reviewed by an experienced MT before being released to the client. That will remain in place until you get the hang of things.

Navigating the Quality Assessment Process

Let's go, quality, let's go! (Stomp, stomp.) Everyone in medical transcription agrees quality is important; however, achieving it is neither simple nor painless. Sometimes it's downright controversial. Understanding the process from both sides can help you navigate it more smoothly.

There are numerous ways of saying that quality matters. Here are some quality-related terms you're likely to come across:

✔ **Quality assurance (QA):** A process put in place to ensure that reports returned to the client are accurately transcribed.

✔ **Quality assessment or review (QA or QR):** Examination of a particular MT's completed reports to assess work quality.

✔ **Quality assessment/review score (QAS or QRS):** A numeric score assigned to an MT that indicates accuracy rate (for example, 98 percent).

✔ **Quality assurance/assessment/review editor (QAE, QRE, or just QE):** The person who performs the quality assessment or review.

The QA process is overseen by senior MTs, who fill in blanks others MTs couldn't, check submitted reports for accuracy and proper formatting, and make corrections. They also may assign grades to individual MTs.

There are three ways a report can end up in QA:

✔ An MT with a problematic report can route it through a QA editor for help. This is called putting the report "on hold" for QA.

✔ All work from a particular MT or for a specific client account can automatically be routed through QA.

✔ Many companies perform random QA audits on an ongoing basis. Periodically (for example, monthly), a sampling of the MT's transcribed reports are spot-checked.

A newly hired MT can expect to be put on 100 percent QA at first. That means every single report is put "on hold" for review by a QE before it is released to the client. When the QE is confident that the new MT is consistently achieving accurate and properly formatted reports, the MT is taken off 100 percent QA.

Making it through the break-in period and graduating from full QA is an accomplishment to be proud of. Going forward, your reports will go to QA only if you send them there, or as part of a random audit. To ensure ongoing quality, many employers conduct periodic assessments of MT work. Periodically, a random sample of reports will be pulled, inspected, and assigned a quality score. The scores of all the reports in the sample are averaged together to come up with an overall score. MTs who exceed a target threshold (for example, 98 percent) sometimes receive a pay bonus; those who fall below may face line rate deduction and/or be put back on more regular QA.

The QA process varies widely among transcription employers. Some are more methodical about it than others. Some assign formal QA scores using a preset scoring framework; others simply mark reports with corrections and return them to the MT for review. Some factor QA scores into pay calculations; others simply draw a line in the sand: Be on the right side of it within a specified period of time or be gone.

For an explanation of how MT pay is calculated and how quality scores can figure in, turn to Chapter 3.

Quality assessment scores, AHDI style

Analyzing documents for accuracy and coming up with a definitive number like 98 percent is no easy thing. For starters, all errors are not equal: Inserting an unnecessary hyphen is trivial in comparison to transcribing a medication name incorrectly. Similarly, using *there* instead of *their* may not endanger a patient, but it's still an error. Factoring all that into generating a consistent and meaningful final score can get tricky fast.

The Association for Healthcare Documentation Integrity (AHDI) took on the challenge and developed a recommended quality-scoring framework. The initial version, in place since about 2005, was replaced with a shiny new system in 2010. The 2010 revision greatly simplified the system. It also takes the sting out of minor punctuation issues.

Key points of the AHDI scoring system include the following:

✔ **Every transcribed document starts with a score of 100.** Points are then deducted to derive a final score.

✔ **Errors are assigned to one of three categories.** The categories are: critical (3-point deduction), noncritical (1-point deduction), or feedback and educational opportunities (no deduction).

✔ **If the same error is repeated multiple times in a document, it's counted only once.**

Thus:

100 − (# of critical errors × 3 points) − (# of noncritical errors × 1 point) = score

A score of 98 or better is considered passing. Because a critical error results in a 3-point deduction, a report containing a critical error automatically fails (100 − 3 = 97).

The AHDI provides detailed guidelines for this system in a whitepaper available in the "Best Practices and Standard Guidelines" section of its website (www.ahdionline.org). The whitepaper provides examples of critical versus noncritical errors, along with a list of items that should not result in point deductions. It also includes example worksheets for QA use.

Understanding the challenges

As reasonable as the pursuit of perfection sounds, in practice, the QA process can get pretty bumpy. By and large, new MTs are very thankful that someone (QA) has their back, but it's not always smooth sailing.

The quality editor and the MT, both of whom are striving to do their jobs well and quickly, can end up butting heads over what should be counted as an error or how serious an error really is. It's unfortunate, because their ultimate goal is the same: accurate and clear medical reports produced in a timely fashion.

Understanding what the QA process is like from both perspectives will put you in a much better position to handle either side of the process you find yourself on.

From the perspective or the MT undergoing QA:

- ✔ Nobody enjoys receiving criticism, and the line between feedback and criticism can be pretty fuzzy.

- ✔ Time spent reviewing QA feedback is unpaid time, as is any time not spent actively transcribing.

- ✔ In some cases, an error is clearly obvious to both sides, but many times what is considered an error can seem arbitrary or unreasonably petty. The latter can quickly lead to hard feelings — as in, are we in this together or is it me vs. you?

- ✔ The MT is most likely trying very hard to do the best job possible. The QA process can feel like a method of punishment rather than a tool for improvement.

From the QA editor's perspective:

- ✔ QA is responsible for preventing mistakes from reaching the client; it's better to err on the side of caution.

- ✔ Like other MTs, most quality editors also are paid on production. It takes a lot more time to "teach" someone than it does to just make corrections. In addition, filling in blanks that seem unwarranted and fixing what appear to be basic mistakes takes time (and can get on a person's nerves).

- ✔ A QE's job is to identify and address errors. If a QE isn't finding any (everyone knows there are occasional mistakes because nobody is perfect), then the QE's own job performance may be questioned.

Challenging a quality assessment penalty

A quality assessment score isn't automatically a take-it-or-leave-it proposition. If you feel you've been improperly dinged, you can appeal. First, however, give yourself a cooling-off period. Wait at least 24 hours before challenging a score. Use that time to evaluate whether the discrepancy is significant enough to be worth your time and energy to dispute. If the effect is minor, sometimes just letting it slide is the more prudent (and cost-effective) option.

If you decide to challenge a QA assessment, the best route is usually to approach your immediate supervisor rather than the QA person directly. Your supervisor most likely has the power to retroactively change a score. Plus, if the supervisor agrees with you, they'll probably pass it on to the QE; if they don't, the QE may never know you disputed, thus avoiding potentially hard feelings on the QE's part.

Be very matter of fact about it, and back up your case with supporting evidence. Here are some possibilities:

- ✔ Citing a specific page from AHDI's *Book of Style for Medical Transcription* is ideal.
- ✔ Referencing previous QA feedback you received, preferably on a report for the same client account, can be powerful.
- ✔ If it's a matter of account specifics that deviate from standard guidelines, the QE may be unaware of the deviation. Pointing that out will clear things up immediately.

Punctuation tends to be a hot button. Getting dinged for something like an allegedly misplaced comma is especially frustrating. In such cases, it can be more effective to argue that your punctuation choice didn't impact the meaning of the sentence rather than argue about whether it was technically correct.

If your employer is calculating a QA score using an error points system, there's a good chance they're using one defined by the AHDI. The AHDI completely made over its recommended scoring system in 2010 (see the "Quality assessment scores, AHDI style" sidebar, earlier in this chapter). Many minor items that resulted in a score deduction under the old system don't under the new one. If your QA report includes fractional points (for example, 1.5 or 0.25) it's probably based on the old system. Alerting your employer about the update may work in your favor, if not immediately then on future evaluations.

Whether your appeal succeeds or is turned down, accept the judgment in a professional manner. Remember that the QE is another MT, like you, who is working hard, occasionally has bad days, and is sticking by what she believes is correct. If you're consistently butting heads with QA, then you'll have to decide whether it's something you can live with or if it may be time to seek a different employer (and a different QE).

HIPAA and Patient Privacy: What You Need to Know

As an MT, you'll be entrusted with sensitive patient data. You have a legal, moral, and ethical duty to protect it. Besides, it's the right thing to do.

Legally speaking, you won't get very far down the MT trail before you run into HIPAA (pronounced hip-uh). HIPAA is an acronym for the Health Insurance Portability and Accountability Act of 1996. The key component that MTs must be up on is the Privacy Rule. That's the part that defines a set of national standards for protection and disclosure of certain types of individual health information, called protected health information (PHI). In a nutshell, if PHI gets out in violation of the Privacy Rule, heads will roll.

Understanding HIPAA regulations

This section is a boiled-down, summary of key information extracted from hundreds of pages of legislation. It's intended to give you the big picture, not a definitive legal determination about how HIPAA applies to you. If you want the full snoozer version, go to www.hhs.gov/ocr/privacy.

HIPAA is a federal statute that made sweeping changes to healthcare laws. Although it was enacted in 1996, it wasn't fully implemented until 2003. Since then, additional laws have been passed that modified regulations and added enforcement provisions.

HIPAA's primary purpose was to help workers continue health insurance coverage when they change jobs or become unemployed. It also included another section, called Administration Simplification (AS), which is the part that has substantially impacted the medical transcription profession. The AS section of HIPAA gives patients greater control of (and access to) their own medical records and how their personal health information is used. That form you now sign every time you visit a new health provider confirming that they've given you a copy of their patient privacy policy comes from this section. It also includes the Privacy Rule and the Security Rule, which together regulate how particular members of the healthcare industry must manage individual health information. You can think of it as the who, what, how, and "or else" of protecting personal health information.

The Privacy Rule applies to all PHI, including paper and electronic. The Security Rule deals specifically with standards for the security of electronic protected health information (e-PHI). It defines administrative, physical, and technical safeguards that must be employed.

Failure to comply with HIPAA can lead to stiff penalties. Civil penalties go from $100 per violation to $25,000 per calendar year, and criminal penalties top out at ten years' imprisonment and a $250,000 fine. Now that's an "or else" with some teeth to it!

HIPAA laws apply to

- ✔ Health plans
- ✔ Healthcare clearinghouses (entities that facilitate handling electronic healthcare transactions)

✔ Healthcare providers who transmit health information in electronic form for certain types of transactions, such as submitting insurance claims

✔ Business associates of the preceding (potentially including you)

The first three are collectively referred to as *covered entities. Business associates* is a term used to described third parties that covered entities disclose PHI to, such as medical transcription services.

Before a covered entity can disclose PHI to a business associate, there must be a written contract in place that ensures the associate will appropriately safeguard the information. The contract is called a *business associate agreement,* and MTs who contract with medical transcription service organizations (MTSOs) can expect to sign one.

Originally, business associates were accountable to the covered entity through these contracts, and the covered entity was accountable to the federal government for HIPAA compliance. The Health Information Technology for Economic and Clinical Health (HITECH) Act, passed in 2009, included provisions that made business associates directly liable to the government for HIPAA violations.

The Privacy Rule and Security Rule are enforced by the Office of Civil Rights (OCR). In 2010, the OCR issued a Notice of Proposed Rulemaking (NPRM) that expands the definition of *business associate* to include subcontractors, a category that includes MT independent contractors (ICs) who work for MTSOs. The NPRM potentially makes MT ICs directly liable to the federal government for failure to comply with HIPAA regulations.

In summary, HIPAA + HITECH + NPRM = MT ICs must preserve, protect, and defend the privacy and confidentiality of the records (voice files, transcribed reports, logs, and so on) handled during the transcription process, and prevent theft or loss of protected health information.

If you're aching for further, intricate details, visit the following websites:

✔ The health information privacy information website of the U.S. Department of Health and Human Services provides extensive information about the HIPAA Privacy Rule and Security Rule. It also includes business associate contract examples. Go to `www.hhs.gov/ocr/privacy/hipaa/understanding/index.html` for more information.

✔ For an overview of HIPAA from the big-picture perspective, not just the patient privacy components, Wikipedia is a good place to start. Go to `http://en.wikipedia.org/wiki/Health_Insurance_Portability_and_Accountability_Act`.

HIPAA is a federal law, but it doesn't override state laws regarding patient privacy. Some states have different laws regulating patient privacy. It's best to be aware of both and comply with the most stringent requirements.

Safeguarding patient privacy

HIPAA or no HIPAA, all MTs have an ethical and moral responsibility to protect patient confidentiality. It's part of the job description. There are some steps you should routinely take as part of handling patient data in a professional matter:

✔ **Don't talk about reports you've transcribed.** Exchanging tidbits of non-identifiable information is acceptable, but never include any details that may identify the patient, even indirectly.

✔ **Put away sensitive data when you leave your work area or when someone else enters it.** That includes not leaving a report in progress up on your computer screen where someone passing by may see it. Enabling password protection on your screensaver can help with this.

✔ **Don't retain patient data any longer than necessary.** Wipe it from your computer hard drive, shred it, or otherwise securely dispose of it as soon as you no longer need it. If you're required to retain something, such as a transcription log, secure it by locking it in a filing cabinet or password-protected location.

✔ **Password-protect your computer, even if it's in your home.** Password-cracking software is very good at guessing passwords, so don't just use your cousin's dog's name. A secure password is at least six characters long, includes uppercase and lowercase letters, includes punctuation marks and/or numbers, and isn't listed in any dictionary. Don't publish your carefully crafted password by attaching it to your computer monitor with a sticky note. Write it down somewhere, but not somewhere anyone can easily get his hands on it.

✔ **If you change computers, securely erase the hard drive on the old one before handing it over to a recycling facility or handing it down to a relative.** Use a secure-erase utility or reformat the drive entirely. Simply deleting sensitive files isn't enough, because deleted data is easy to recover by those in the know.

✔ **Protect your computer from Internet-based hackers with firewall and antivirus software.** For added protection, shut down your computer when you're not using it. When it's not on, there's no way anyone from the Internet can break in, no matter how clever she is.

✔ **Lock your laptop and keep security in mind when you take it on the road.** If someone breaks into your residence or hotel room and makes off with it, they may well walk off with PHI in addition to your valuable laptop. You can buy cable locks that enable you to securely fasten a laptop to a work surface.

If you're working from home, don't let the relaxed surroundings lull you into a false sense of security. The world is an unpredictable place; hackers, burglars, and Mother Nature are just a few of the forces you can't control. You can, however, take steps to protect the personal and confidential information entrusted to you.

Chapter 17

Climbing the Career Ladder

. . . .

. . . .

Many medical transcriptionists (MTs) are quite satisfied to settle in and work from home transcribing and/or editing medical reports, thank you very much! Others feel the urge to branch out. Even if you're not planning to expand or change your job role, it's important to maintain and hone your MT skills and take an active role in your profession. If you're the ambitious type, you'll need to be extra attentive to staying at the top of your game so that you can reach your next goal as quickly as possible.

In this chapter, you explore career path options and ways to nourish and grow your MT career. You find out how and where to take advantage of professional development opportunities that will help you keep up with the new technologies, medications, and procedures that arrive every day. You also discover the benefits of joining a professional organization and which ones to consider. Getting certified can be both professionally and personally rewarding, and this chapter helps you decide if certification is a path you want to take. Finally, I end this chapter with tips to keep in mind when changing employers so that you can make that potentially delicate process go smoothly.

Mapping Out Common Career Paths

As you build experience, you'll gain access to additional job roles. The first step is to take on more complex report types and client accounts. When you hit full stride, those additional doors will begin to open, including the following:

✔ After you've mastered the secrets of deciphering difficult dictation and applying obscure formatting rules, you may decide to become a Quality assurance (QA) editor. QA editors audit transcribed reports to make sure they're completely accurate.

✔ If taking a leadership role appeals to you, consider stepping into a team leader or supervisory position. Team leaders and supervisors provide guidance on exactly how things should be done for a particular transcription client and help fill in especially tricky blanks.

✔ If you have entrepreneurial tendencies, you may want to explore running your own transcription business. That may mean starting one from scratch or taking charge of an existing medical transcription service organization (MTSO).

✔ Truly seasoned MTs can move into teaching and mentoring, working in online MT schools and community colleges.

As your career progresses, you'll meet people who've done all these things. They'll be your supervisors, teachers, and employers. While getting to know them, you'll also get a taste of what their work entails. If you get itchy for a career move, tap them as resources to help you decide where to go next.

Keeping Current through Continuing Education

You'll pick up new medical knowledge every day, just by virtue of working as an MT. If you're like many MTs, you're a passionate learner, and you're going to want even more than you learn on the job. Fortunately, getting that medical or technical education fix is easier than ever. Courses and seminars are available to help you

✔ Get acquainted with the latest technologies, such as electronic health records (EHRs)

✔ Learn new productivity techniques

✔ Tune up your speech-recognition editing skills

✔ Study up on Health Insurance Portability and Accountability Act (HIPAA) compliance and patient privacy regulations

✔ Bone up on a specific medical specialty

✔ Explore potential career paths

✔ Prepare for a certification exam

Where to find courses and seminars

The quickest route to continuing education is directly through your computer. Taking an online course from the comfort of your desk (or anywhere else you can get an Internet connection) is easy. Online training options include the following:

- **Webinars:** These are single-session presentations, typically an hour long. A webinar can be prerecorded or live. A big plus of live webinars is that often you can ask questions and interact with other students.

- **Online courses:** These include multiple sessions or lessons and go into a subject in depth. Most online courses are self-paced. You can log on and learn any time you want, although there's usually a limit on how long you have to complete the course. An online course may include access to an instructor via e-mail.

  A growing number of online courses incorporate remote access to the technology or tools you're learning about. That means you can log on to someone else's hardware and software and get hands-on experience without having to travel anywhere or invest in your own materials. Talk about handy!

As convenient as online training is, face-to-face learning is hard to beat if you have access to it and can work it into your schedule. Unlike online training, you have to show up where the presenter does, but the payoff is that you get to interact with other people live and in person. Classroom options include the following:

- **Seminars:** These usually last a half or full day.

- **Formal courses:** You can find courses through a nearby community college.

- **Annual Convention and Expo (ACE):** This event is put on by the Association for Healthcare Documentation Integrity (AHDI). It offers a smorgasbord of learning and networking opportunities.

When you're ready to start continuing your education, the AHDI website (www.ahdionline.org) is a good place to start picking through options. You also can search the web for "medical transcription continuing education." If you're really lucky, there will be a local MT group in your area that brings in presenters from time to time.

How to fund your ongoing learning

If you're like most MTs, you'll have to pay for ongoing training out of your own pocket. If you're working as an employee rather than as an independent contractor, hitting up your employer for a subsidy is always worth a shot. When you ask, be sure to specify how the fact that you're taking the course will benefit your employer.

Once you get some experience under your belt, there's another option: Trade. If you make a presentation or volunteer your time to set up, clean up, or help manage a seminar or conference, you often can attend the event for free.

If you do have to foot the bill yourself, you may be able to recoup some of your expenses by taking advantage of tax breaks. Your options are tied to your employment status:

- ✔ **Employee:** If you itemize deductions on your federal tax return, you may be able to claim a deduction for qualifying work-related education expenses on Schedule A. If the training involves an overnight stay away from home, you can most likely deduct part of your travel, meals, and lodging expenses too.

- ✔ **Independent contractor:** As a self-employed person, you can deduct qualifying education-related expenses directly from your income, just as you would any other business expense. This will feed through your Schedule C along with virtually everything else.

Check IRS Publication 970, "Tax Benefits for Education" (`www.irs.gov/pub/irs-pdf/p970.pdf`), for the what and how of deducting work-related education expenses. (Look for the section titled "Business Deduction for Work-Related Education.") If you hire a professional to do your taxes, be sure to tell him about your education expenditures — he'll know which forms to use.

If you work as an independent contractor, be sure to check out Chapter 17 for additional tips on financial matters specific to freelancers.

Joining Up: Professional Organizations for Medical Transcriptionists

Launching a new career and joining a professional association frequently go hand in hand. Even so, as a new MT, you won't be rolling in the dough, so handing some of it over to a professional group may not be high on your list. There are compelling reasons to do it anyway. Here are just five of the benefits joining up can give you:

✔ You have a way to get involved with your profession, not just work in it.

✔ Your membership ensures the existence of a "voice" for MTs, so they (you!) have a presence at the table when it comes to employers and the government. A collection of voices is much stronger than a single voice. Add yours!

✔ You get ready access to continuing education opportunities (and a push to use them).

✔ You receive a steady supply of newsletters/publications and a chance to participate in insider discussions about the latest developments in the field.

✔ Membership is a résumé builder that shows you're passionate about your profession and ready and willing to participate in its growth and development.

This list doesn't even include the networking opportunities, mentoring possibilities, discounts, and numerous other benefits professional associations typically make available to members.

If you decide a professional membership belongs on your to-do list, your first two stops should be:

✔ Association for Healthcare Documentation Integrity (AHDI)

✔ American Health Information Management Association (AHIMA)

AHDI specifically takes the medical transcriptionist perspective: health data capture and documentation. AHIMA's mission centers around the management of that data. The two subject areas are inextricably intertwined and becoming more so every day. The two organizations are increasingly so as well.

Why more MTs don't join up

So, if professional associations offer all this great stuff, why don't more MTs join up? It comes down to two things: cost and frustration over what they do and don't accomplish. Before you lock down your wallet, though, take a minute to consider whether these may actually be arguments for joining rather than against.

There's no question that it's a challenging time to be an MT. There's tremendous change going on. New opportunities are opening up, including a broad availability of the option to work from home. But there's also a lot of pressure for MTs to produce more, faster, and for less pay; plus, a cloud of uncertainty surrounds the move to EHR. Put them all together and you have MTs who are on a tight budget, many of whom who feel professional organizations like AHDI aren't doing enough to help them ride this wave of change.

Why even consider giving an organization that isn't doing what you want it to some of your limited funds? Reread the list of benefits earlier, especially the first two items on the list.

A student membership is an ideal way to test the waters of a professional organization with minimal commitment. Both AHDI and AHIMA offer inexpensive student memberships. There's an important difference, though: AHDI student membership is open to anyone enrolled in a medical transcription training program, whereas AHIMA only lets in people who are enrolled in a training program that is directly affiliated with AHIMA.

AHDI and AHIMA are in many ways competing for the same membership pool, which, of course, includes you. Given the convergence of their constituencies, it's quite possible they'll end up merging at some point.

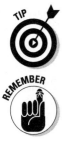

Whether you join one or both of these organizations, you'll gain the most bang for your buck by being active. If you lack the time or inclination to take a hands-on position, consider joining up anyway just to play a supporting role.

Dues paid professional organizations that are related to your business are deductible on your federal income tax return. For employees, that means on Schedule A. For independent contractors, the dues will come under the expenses section of Schedule C.

Association for Healthcare Documentation Integrity

AHDI (www.ahdionline.org) is the central professional association MTs join. If you're going to join just one professional organization, this should be it. Here are a few of AHDI's many accomplishments:

- ✔ It crafted and continues to update a detailed model curriculum for training new medical transcriptionists. The curriculum is freely available through the AHDI website.

- ✔ It develops and disseminates industry best-practices guidelines, including an "MT Bill of Rights" and model job descriptions for MT-related roles.

- ✔ It publishes *The Book of Style for Medical Transcription,* the de-facto standard for formatting medical reports.

- ✔ It puts on an annual conference, ACE, that is a fantastic (if somewhat expensive) opportunity to immerse yourself in all that is MT and the future of MT. *Note:* Some employers pay at least some of the costs of attending ACE, such as the registration fee.

- ✔ It's absolutely packed with leaders who are involved and invested in creating and upholding the highest standards of practice in healthcare documentation and the role MTs play in it. These are people with first-hand experience in the pleasures and pains of MT work.

This organization isn't without controversy, but given what it's had to work with and face, it's done an impressive job so far. If you're looking at the big picture, you should be supporting AHDI.

American Health Information Management Association

AHIMA's area of focus is healthcare data management and medical coding. Although AHIMA (www.ahima.org) isn't specifically an MT-focused association, there's a lot of overlap. The two organizations have worked together on a variety of initiatives, including drafting guidelines defining optimal turnaround times for different types of medical reports.

AHIMA offers professional certifications via its Commission on Certification for Health Informatics and Information Management (CCHIIM). The growing list includes credentials related to health information management, data privacy and security, and clinical documentation improvement.

Getting Certified

There's no particular credential you must have in order to become an MT, but that doesn't mean you can't benefit from earning one after you're on the job. Professional credentials are great motivators. They push you to get and keep current and provide a blueprint for expanding your skills into new areas. They also add a nice sheen to your résumé, and that can translate into a pay increase or greater career mobility.

Certifications and certificates are not the same thing. Certifications are earned by passing exams. Certificates are awarded for completing a course or attending a seminar. Both can add to your résumé, but certifications typically carry more weight.

AHDI offers two certifications for medical transcriptionists:

- **Registered Medical Transcriptionist (RMT):** For new graduates, specialty MTs, and MTs working up to taking the CMT exam

- **Certified Medical Transcriptionist (CMT):** For experienced MTs with two or more years of acute-care or multi-specialty transcription

You can either earn the RMT and then progress to the CMT or take the all-in-one Credential Qualifying Exam (CQE) that covers the material from both.

For more information on the RMT and CMT exams, turn to Chapter 4.

Switching Employers the Right Way

People change employers for many reasons. Even if you're fortunate enough to land a starting position that's a perfect match at the time you accept it, your needs and interests may subsequently change. You may find that you want to

- ✔ Change from employee to independent contractor or vice versa

- ✔ Perform a different kind of transcription, perhaps moving from clinic to acute care work or into a particular specialty

- ✔ Seek out an employer who offers higher pay or a better schedule

- ✔ Move on from an employment arrangement you simply don't like

Whatever the reason, there are a few important things to keep in mind as you undertake a move. Underlying all of them is the importance of thinking long-term and maintaining your best professional persona every step of the way. Of particular note are the following:

- ✔ **Consider whether your issue can be addressed without switching employers.** Do you really want to start from scratch elsewhere? It's possible a different schedule, account, or supervisor would square things away for you. This is a discussion you should schedule rather than rush into — that way, whoever you're approaching will (hopefully) have set aside time to talk. The odds for a successful resolution rocket upward when both sides remain calm, cool, and collected and have time to think about options.

- ✔ **If you decide a switch is in order, conduct a patient and methodical job search before making it.** Leaving an existing employment arrangement only to find yourself in another one that isn't what you want either is all too common.

- ✔ **Don't quit your current position until you've landed a new one, and then give your current employer two weeks' notice before making the switch.** Leaving abruptly is unprofessional and unfair. Your current employer deserves the opportunity to transition your work to another MT. Your new employer will respect you for it.

- ✔ **Be tactful when giving your reason for leaving, even if you're really aggravated with your soon-to-be-former employer.** Disparaging remarks, even when true, can brand you as complainer or, at the very least, unprofessional. It's much better to say you're looking for new opportunities, an alternate work schedule, or different work types. One or more of those will be true anyway. The employer you're leaving will want to know why, too. Exercise similar tact. The future is unpredictable, and you never know who you may run into down the road.

Although few people, if any, find a job hunt fun, the results can certainly justify the effort. If it's time to move on, do it — but take the time to do it well.

Chapter 18

Working from Home

• •

In This Chapter

▶ Connecting to the Internet

▶ Considering your computer options

▶ Picking out transcription gear

▶ Taking technical support personally

▶ Fending off distractions and well-intentioned neighbors

• •

*T*he opportunity to work from home is brought to us by the wonders of computer technology; so are a lot of potential headaches. Getting a firm grip on what equipment you'll need and features to look for will help you maximize the wonders and minimize the headaches.

The first thing a home-based medical transcriptionist (MT) needs is a suitable workspace. A room with a door you can close is ideal, but an organized corner will do. Pick a spot that has enough space for your computer, reference books, and a comfortable chair. The farther it is from the busiest areas of your home, the better.

Technically speaking, you'll need the following:

✔ An Internet connection

✔ A desktop or laptop computer running Microsoft Windows

✔ Transcription software, installed on your computer or on a remote server you connect to

✔ A foot pedal for controlling dictation playback

✔ Headphones

✔ A plan for protecting your equipment and managing technical troubles that may arise

A large part of optimal MT workspace design comes down to how you set up the furnishings and computer equipment. Chapter 20 addresses the ins and outs of selecting furniture and arranging your gear with health and comfort in mind.

Staying Connected: Internet Service

There are many ways you can bring Internet service to your home. The most popular are cable, DSL, and satellite. Forget about dial-up — it's just too slow to be accepted by MT employers anymore.

- ✔ **Cable:** Cable Internet uses the same coaxial cable that delivers cable TV programming. It offers the fastest connection speed and is very reliable.

- ✔ **DSL:** DSL is short for *digital subscriber line.* DSL service is delivered over standard telephone lines. It's usually slower than cable but faster than satellite. Neighborhoods that have been outfitted with fiber-optic phone lines can obtain much higher speeds. ADSL (asymmetric digital subscriber line) is a form of DSL.

- ✔ **Satellite:** Satellite Internet is usually the slowest and most expensive type of connection. However, if you live in a remote location, it may be your only option. To use it, you'll need a satellite dish installed on the exterior of your home.

High-speed wireless is starting to appear in some major metropolitan areas. Due to its limited availability and the tight restrictions wireless providers set on the amount of data you can transfer, it isn't well suited for MT work yet.

Choosing an Internet connection type is a matter of weighing availability, price, speed, and reliability. When picking a plan, keep in mind what else will be going on in your home (and on your Internet connection) while you're working. If you'll be sharing the connection with others who will be streaming movies or playing games at the same time, you'll need a higher-capacity connection.

 Wired connections are significantly faster than Wi-Fi ones. It's worth finding a discreet way to run a cable from your Internet modem to your computer. Network cables are just like phone cables, with a jack on each end; plug one end into the modem or router and the other into your computer's networking (Ethernet) port. If you're sharing your Internet connection with other computers, some can be wired and others wireless if you have a router that allows it.

Choosing a Computer Setup

If you take a job as an employee, your employer may ship you a computer preloaded with software and ready to go. However, that's increasingly rare, and many MTs work from a computer they own. If you already have a computer that's only a few years old (say, four years or less) it'll likely be up to the task. However, even if you already own a computer that you could work from, there are some pretty good reasons to have a computer you dedicate to MT work and nothing else:

- ✔ If you're an independent contractor (IC), as many MTs are, a computer you purchase strictly for work will be tax deductible.

- ✔ Private health information needs to stay private — it's legally required (see Chapter 16). Separating business and personal computing makes it easier to accomplish this.

- ✔ The more web surfing and game playing that's done on your computer, the more likely it will become infected with a virus or malware.

- ✔ If you're sharing, other users may inadvertently mess up your stuff.

Laptop or desktop?

MT work can be done from both laptop and desktop computers. Unless you have a compelling reason to use a laptop, a desktop computer is the way to go. You'll have much more control over the arrangement of the various components, and you can set them up for optimum comfort and efficiency.

If you work on a transcription system that's entirely Internet-based, it's likely to have a piece of local "client" software that allows you to securely connect to the remote system, while everything else is located on a central server. It's quite possible that you can install the client software on both your desktop and a laptop, allowing you to work from either one.

Desktops

Here are some advantages of desktops:

- ✔ They're more ergonomically adjustable, because you can move the screen and keyboard independently.

- ✔ They allow for greater productivity potential for the same reasons.

- ✔ They're easier to upgrade and expand.

- ✔ They offer more places to plug stuff in (and there's always more stuff to plug in).

- ✔ You have more options when selecting monitors, keyboards, and other peripherals.

If you're short on desk space, an all-in-one desktop may be tempting. Standard desktops consist of a case that holds the computing components and a separate monitor. All-in-ones integrate computing components and the display into a single unit, resulting in a computer that has fewer cables and takes up less space. However, all-in-ones don't offer the performance and flexibility of a desktop computer or the portability of a laptop computer, making them a less desirable option.

Laptops

The main advantage of laptops is portability. You can work from virtually anywhere you can get an Internet connection.

On the downside:

- The smaller keyboard and screen size and lack of ability to adjust the components independently will reduce your productivity and comfort.

- You have very limited ability to upgrade components or add new technology.

- Laptops have a tendency to overheat when used continuously for long periods, which can contribute to a shorter computer lifespan.

If you decide to go with a laptop as your primary work computer, get an external full-sized keyboard. An external monitor is also a good idea. Almost all laptops include ports for connecting both. If you think you'll be plugging and unplugging them often, consider getting a docking station; it makes connecting a laptop to a set of external devices as simple as plugging in a single USB cable. That makes it easy to bring a lot of desktop features to your laptop, including external monitor, keyboard, speakers, and extra USB ports, while still allowing you to unplug and go when you want.

Specs: Operating system, hard drive, and RAM

Medical transcription work requires a lot of brain power but not a lot of computing power. There's no real need for a high-end CPU, super video card, or gobs of storage (unless you want them for another purpose), and money you save there can be put toward a better (or additional) monitor or cushy chair.

The specifications suggested here are guidelines provided to help you get the performance you need without paying for things you don't. Given the pace of technological change, it's possible an inflatable, gerbil-powered supercomputer costing $99.95 will hit the market the day after this book is published. If so, you'll probably want to give it a look — it would be a fun thing to have on your desk.

Before going computer shopping, arm yourself with a little terminology so salespeople can't overwhelm you with geek-speak. Here are the terms you need to know:

- ✔ **CPU:** The central processing unit (processor) is an electronic chip that serves as the brain of the computer.

- ✔ **RAM:** Random access memory is the computer equivalent to human working memory, where things are briefly stored and constantly swapped in and out.

- ✔ **Motherboard:** A flat circuit board (usually weird green) inside the computer that everything else plugs into, including the CPU and RAM. It's like the interstate highway system for your computer. Motherboards contain slots for plugging in smaller circuit boards, such as a graphics card.

- ✔ **Card:** A small circuit board you can plug into the motherboard to add an additional feature, such as enhanced sound or graphics.

- ✔ **Port:** An opening where you plug something in, like a monitor, keyboard, network cable, or transcription foot pedal. There are different kinds of ports for plugging in different devices.

- ✔ **Hard drive:** The primary storage device where all your files and data that need to be kept longer than a few seconds are stored.

- ✔ **Bluetooth:** A wireless technology for exchanging data over very short distances, such as between a keyboard and a computer. It can also be used to sync information between devices, such as between a cellphone and a computer. It's not the only short-range wireless technology, but it's increasingly common.

There's plenty more jargon where this came from, but don't sweat the extra alphabet soup. Defining it all would require an entire, very dull dictionary, and most of it just isn't that important to the average computer user. If you run across a stumper term you're concerned about, Google and your nearest computer salesperson stand ready to define it for you.

Desktops and laptops come with basic sound and graphics capabilities built in. If you want higher-level performance, you can add on a specialized graphics or sound card. Technical specifications for a desktop and laptop computers are listed in Table 18-1.

Microsoft Windows is the operating system of choice for medical transcription. As of Windows 7, it's available in 32-bit and 64-bit versions. The "bit" thing has to do with how it handles data, not how many pieces it comes in. A computer running 32-bit Windows will work fine, but if you're buying new, go with 64-bit, or you may end up upgrading later.

Table 18-1	Computer Specifications for MTs	
Component	**Desktop Specifications**	**Laptop Specifications**
CPU	Don't worry about this. The CPU in any new desktop will be sufficient.	Don't worry about this. The CPU in any new laptop will be sufficient.
RAM	At least 4GB.	At least 4GB.
Hard drive	At least 250GB.	At least 250GB, with 7200 rpm.
Graphics	The built-in graphics capabilities of any budget system will suffice, but consider adding a graphics card for better performance and so you can connect multiple monitors.	The built-in graphics capabilities of any budget laptop will suffice.
Sound	Nothing special required.	Nothing special required.
Networking	Built-in Ethernet networking (looks like an oversized telephone wall jack). Add a wireless networking card if you'll be using wireless Internet connection.	Built-in Ethernet and Wi-Fi networking. 802-11n.
Bluetooth	Less common on desktops than laptops but worth considering if it adds only minimally to the overall cost. If you want to connect wireless external devices, like a keyboard or mouse, a USB port can be used instead. If you want to wirelessly sync data to a tablet or cellphone, then Bluetooth is a good option to get. You can also easily add Bluetooth later with a USB adapter.	Not a must-have, but Bluetooth capability will enable you to connect external devices like a keyboard and mouse without using a USB port to do it (as long as the devices also support Bluetooth). Comes built-in to many laptops.
Display	See "Monitors: How to choose," later in this chapter.	15-inch to 17-inch display with matte finish. Avoid wide-screen displays (see "Monitors: How to choose," later in this chapter).
Other features	As many USB ports as possible (minimum of four), with at least two of them on the front of the computer for easy access. DVD drive with read/write capability.	As many USB ports as possible; many laptops come with two, but more is better. DVD drive with read/write capability. Ports for plugging in an external keyboard, monitor, and mouse.

When comparing computers, pay special attention to:

- ✔ **RAM:** The amount of RAM you have matters, because swapping things in and out of RAM is much faster than reading and writing to a hard drive, which is what happens when RAM is full. Since MTs often have multiple applications running simultaneously, RAM should be high on your priority list. Of note, 32-bit versions of Windows can't take advantage of more than 4GB, but 64-bit versions can.

- ✔ **USB ports:** USB stands for _universal serial bus,_ a type of connection used to connect external devices to a computer. You can't have too many USB ports — they're currently the top connection type for plugging in new stuff. Things that typically plug into a USB port include keyboards, mice/trackballs, printers, external hard drives, and most transcription foot pedals.

- ✔ **Graphics:** Whatever graphics processor comes built into your computer will do, but if you add a graphics card, you'll get much better performance for activities like watching videos. Most important, pay attention to the number of graphics ports you can connect a monitor to. A desktop computer should have at least two of them. You may not use both right off the bat, but if you stick with MT work, you're likely to want to hook up a second monitor.

You may be wondering about sound capabilities; after all, you're going to be listening to a lot of dictation audio on this computer. From the computer specs perspective, the integrated sound provided on typical motherboard should do the job fine. Some MTs opt to install a dedicated sound card and are thrilled with the results. Usually, though, unintelligible dictation is a result of something other than the quality of your sound system.

Monitors: How to choose?

When monitor shopping, the sheer amount of variables can be daunting; however, for those of us who aren't video editors or big-time gamers, most of them aren't important. Here are the key things to pay attention to:

- ✔ **Connection type:** The monitor connection type must be the same as the graphics port on your computer. DVI is the current standard, but if you have an older desktop or laptop it may only have a connection for a VGA monitor. It doesn't really matter what the acronyms mean, only that the monitor and the port you plug it into share the same one.

- ✔ **Size:** Monitor size is measured diagonally and runs from 15 to 30 inches. Many MTs find 17 to 22 inches a good size. After a certain point, bigger can actually become a drawback unless you have a particular need for it. Larger monitors cost more and take up more desk space. They also stretch information all the way across the screen, so you'll have to constantly resize document windows to get a comfortable reading width. If your goal is to view multiple documents or program windows simultaneously, two smaller monitors tends to be a better solution than one huge one.

Using two monitors instead of one is a big productivity booster. The best part: It's really easy to set up. Chapter 9 reveals all.

✔ **Resolution:** Resolution defines how many pixels can be displayed on a screen. For example, a monitor with 1920 x 1080 resolution can display 1920 pixels across and 1080 from top to bottom. The higher the resolution, the more information can be displayed on the screen. That does come with a tradeoff; although the objects on the screen will be sharp, they'll be smaller, which can contribute to eye strain.

✔ **Adjustable base:** Pick a monitor that allows you to easily tilt and swivel the screen. It' surprising how many monitors lack this basic but crucial feature. Height adjustability is a big plus, though you can accomplish the same thing with a thick book if necessary.

✔ **Additional niceties:**

  • Monitors with built-in speakers can save desk space and reduce cable clutter. They're not going to offer symphony sound quality, but neither do standard desktop speakers. Mostly you'll be using headphones anyway.

  • Some monitors come with additional USB ports built in. If you've already got plenty, don't worry about it, but if you're short, it's an easy way to get more.

What to watch out for:

✔ Avoid screens with a glossy finish; they make colors look sharper but add a lot of glare. Matte-finish screens are a lot gentler on your eyes.

✔ Be careful not to buy a wide-screen monitor by mistake. Many people don't realize that the increased width comes with decreased height. Wide screens are good for watching videos and graphics but not so good when it comes to working with documents, because the vertical space is shorter, making less of the document visible at once.

Keyboard

There's no "right" MT keyboard, and what's ideal for one MT can feel awkward to another. If possible, try out multiple keyboards before making a decision. Office superstores and electronics outlets are great places to get hands-on experience before you pick "the one."

Ergonomic keyboards are designed to align your wrists and hands in a more natural, theoretically carpal-tunnel-resistant position. They do so by splitting the keys down the middle and angling the halves slightly outward. Many people find them more comfortable, but people with narrow shoulders may find a standard rectangular keyboard works better.

Here are the features to consider:

✔ Cursor keys arranged in an upside-down T configuration (with the up arrow positioned above the other three keys) are more intuitive and comfortable to use than cursor keys arranged in a straight row.

✔ Some keyboards include extra keys that perform common functions, like turning speaker volume up and down. It seems like such a small thing, but it adds a lot of convenience. In some cases the keys are programmable, so you can create a multi-part macro, assign it to one of the keys, and execute it with a single tap.

Mouse or trackball

Your computer needs a pointer device of some kind — a mouse, trackball, or, for a laptop, a built-in touchpad. Ideally you'll be keeping your hands on your keyboard and making only minimal use of the pointing device, so the details aren't as important as other aspects of your setup. Nonetheless, here are some tips to keep in mind:

✔ Ergonomic mice and trackballs are much more comfortable to use. Lefties, you may be living in a righty world, but there are pointing devices specifically designed for you.

✔ If your work surface is limited in size, consider a trackball. They stay in one spot, so there's no mouse pad or extra desk space required.

Scoping Out Transcription Gear

Every MT needs a transcription foot pedal and a set of high-quality headphones. You can transcribe without them in a pinch, but transcribing with one hand tied behind your back would probably be faster.

Headphones

Headphones provide much better sound quality than computer speakers and help block out surrounding noise. Don't try to use headphones from an MP3 player or other device, because those are optimized for music, not human speech. Headphones made specifically for transcription will give you a fighting chance at understanding what that mumbling dictator is really saying.

Transcription headphones start at less than $20 and go as high as you're willing to pay. Figure 18-1 shows the two basic styles. Standard transcription headphones have soft foam or rubber cushions that fit comfortably in the ears and a very lightweight frame that hangs below the chin.

MTs who find background noise problematic can opt for noise-cancelling headphones. They go over top of your head like traditional headphones and cover your ears entirely. Instead of physically blocking out external noise, they use a sophisticated electronic feedback system to counteract it, effectively making it disappear. Even seemingly minor sounds, like the clicking of keys on a loud keyboard, can get on your nerves over time. These headphones can make them disappear. As you've probably guessed, noise-cancelling headphones cost substantially more than a basic transcription headset.

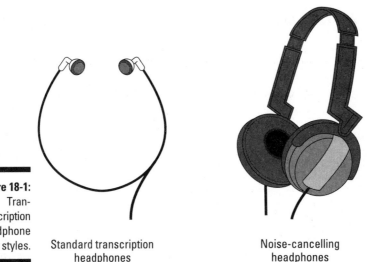

Figure 18-1:
Transcription headphone styles.

Standard transcription headphones

Noise-cancelling headphones

Headphones come in traditional (analog) and USB versions. Analog headphones have a 3.5mm plug that plugs into an audio jack on your computer. USB headphones connect to a USB port instead. Either type is fine for MT work. The pros and cons of each are summarized in Table 18-2. Whichever type you select, make sure it has a cord that's long enough for your setup; 10 feet or longer will usually do it. Although not a necessity, a volume control incorporated into the cord can come in handy.

Table 18-2	Audio Jack vs. USB Headphones	
	Pros	*Cons*
Audio jack headphones	Very simple: Plug in and go.	Sometimes the audio jack is located in a hard-to-reach spot, like on the back of the computer.
		You may have to unplug another audio device, such as your speakers, to plug them in. Some speakers bypass this problem by adding a second audio jack.
USB head-phones	You can have USB head-set and speakers plugged in at the same time, since they use different jacks.	There's a slight delay between when you plug them in and when they begin to work. Also, if they come unplugged while you're working, you may have to restart the application to get the sound back.
	Your USB port may be located in a position that's easier to reach for plug-ging and unplugging.	They take up a USB port, which are often in short supply.

Foot pedals

A foot pedal (also called a WAV pedal) enables you to control dictation play-back with your toes. You can play, rewind, and fast forward by tapping differ-ent sections of the pedal with the front of your foot.

Foot pedals are differentiated by the type of connector used to plug them into a computer or transcriber device. Figure 18-2 shows a foot pedal and two common connector types, USB and serial. Although most foot pedals look and function similarly, the connector matters because some transcription software will work only with a particular type of connector.

✔ **USB foot pedals** are by far the most widely used. The connector is a small rectangular plug (12mm x 4.5mm) that plugs into a USB port. One edge of the connection is slightly wider than the other, which prevents you from plugging it in upside down.

✔ **Serial foot pedals** use a DB-9 serial connector. The connector is like the letter *D* when viewed head-on and has nine holes. Most new computers don't come with a serial port anymore, because it's old technology, but some transcription services still use software that requires a serial foot pedal. Getting a serial port added to a desktop computer is pretty easy, but it's often impossible for laptops. You may be able to get away with using a USB to DB-9 adapter instead, but you'll be venturing into technically tricky territory.

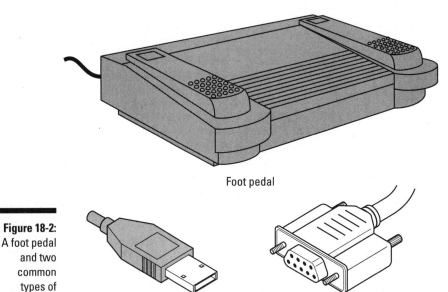

Foot pedal

Figure 18-2:
A foot pedal
and two
common
types of
connectors.

USB connector

Serial connector

In the increasingly rare event that you use a device other than your computer, such as a C-Phone, to play back transcription, it will come with its own foot pedal (with its own special connector type, of course).

Which transcription pedal you'll need is determined by the transcription platform you use. Fortunately, there's a lot of cross-compatibility, especially when it comes to newer USB foot pedals. The best strategy is to continue with the pedal you used during MT training as long as possible. There's no reason to buy another one unless you have to.

MTs often keep a spare backup pedal and headphones on hand, just in case. Some even keep an entire semi-retired computer, too.

Tackling the Technical Details

As a home-based MT, you are your own first line of technical support. If you're an employee, there may be someone you can call for help, but that person may be unavailable when you need her or unable to fix a problem from afar. The more you can do on your own, the better off you'll be. Here are some things you should know for sure:

✔ How to block trouble from entering your computer

✔ How to back up and restore your computer data

✔ Where to get help if you can't solve a problem yourself

Protecting your assets

Computer gear is more reliable than ever, but there are still things that can bring it to its knees in the blink of an eye. Too much electricity, too little electricity, and nefarious individuals are chief among them. Spilling coffee on your keyboard will end badly, too, but you already know how to prevent that.

To protect your equipment, you'll need a surge protector for each wall outlet. Don't even consider going without. Most people think of electricity as an on/off thing, but it's not; it also fluctuates, sometimes substantially. If you've ever noticed your lights flicker, you've witnessed a power fluctuation. When too much electricity comes down the line (a surge) or too little (a brownout or blackout), bad things can happen to your equipment and data. A power surge a brief as one or two nanoseconds can fry your gear.

A basic multi-outlet surge protector, or power strip, contains five or six outlets and provides a small amount of protection. They generally cost $10 to $20. Larger surge protectors, sometimes called *surge stations,* fit on the floor under your desk and provide superior protection. They start at around $30, with more advanced models hitting $100 or more. Neither of these will be any help at all if your power goes out entirely, but a UPS will.

An uninterruptable power supply (UPS) combines surge protection with a battery backup. If power goes out or fluctuates, the battery takes over, and your computer will continue to run uninterrupted. In the case of a complete outage, you'll have a few minutes to save your work and shut down your computer normally. Some UPS units will even gracefully shut down your computer for you. A basic UPS can be had for as little as $50. Prices go up for units that can handle larger power surges and provide longer battery time.

Blocking nefarious individuals requires a different approach. A lot of people seem to have nothing better to do than mess up other people's computers. To avoid becoming a victim, run antivirus software every minute of every day and employ the firewall function built into Microsoft Windows. There are plenty of antivirus programs to choose among, including Microsoft Security Essentials, which you can get for free at `http://windows.microsoft.com/mse`.

Backing up

If your files are wiped out by a virus that manages to sneak through your defenses or you accidentally delete a key document, a lot of time and work can vanish down the drain in seconds. If you've been a wise computer owner and kept regular backups of your data, it becomes an inconvenience instead of a disaster. There's really no excuse for not making regular backups, because these days it's pretty easy to set up an automated backup system that will backup critical files or the entire contents of your computer while you sleep. You can either

- ✔ Install backup software, such as Norton Ghost, that will back up your data to an external drive connected to your computer or home network. Windows 7 and later versions have a built-in backup and restore facility that will do the job, too.

- ✔ Subscribe to an Internet backup service such as Backblaze, Carbonite, or Norton Online Backup, which copies your data to a remote server for storage.

Finding tech support

Sooner or later, things will go awry: Your keyboard will quit working, your computer will slow to a crawl, or your Internet connectivity will vanish, and you're going to have to figure out what to do. If you already have a plan in place you'll be ready to spring into action and get back up and running sooner.

There are two basic elements you can put in place immediately:

- ✔ Make a written copy of critical contact information so you'll have it on hand, not locked away inside a nonfunctional computer. Include names and phone numbers for your employer, supervisor, clients, Internet service provider, power company, child's school and daycare — anyone you may need to notify or contact.

✔ Identify a local computer service location, technical guru, or computer-savvy friend (better yet, all three) you can call for help with issues you can't resolve on your own, and include them on your emergency list.

Before calling in the big (and potentially expensive) guns, take a shot at fixing it yourself. If you're smart enough to handle MT work, you're plenty smart enough to troubleshoot basic computer problems. When a problem is more annoying than catastrophic, there's a good chance you can figure it out yourself. Here are some places to start:

✔ If an application stops responding or your computer locks up, exit any applications you can normally. Then turn off your computer, wait 30 seconds, and turn it on again. This will fix an astonishing array of common problems.

✔ If there's an error message involved, copy it down word-for-word and Google it (with quotes around it). If you can't Google it from your computer, then do it from someone else's.

✔ If your system has slowed to a crawl, close everything and run a full system scan with your antivirus software (you do have it installed and up-to-date, right)? Run a malware scanner like Malewarebytes Anti-Malware, too; it will catch and remove things other programs may miss. Get a copy of the free version now (`www.malwarebytes.org`) and keep it on your desktop. Some malware will block your Internet connection (except for its own nefarious purposes), and this program is absolutely miraculous in restoring it — but only if you've already got it on your computer.

✔ If something just stops working, give every cable that goes in or out of your computer and other equipment a jiggle (at both ends), including network and power cords. Things occasionally work loose, in which case all you have to do is plug them back in and possibly restart your computer.

✔ If your wireless keyboard or mouse starts acting flaky or quits entirely, it probably just needs a new battery.

It's a good idea to pick up a copy of *Windows For Dummies* for the version of Windows you use and keep it on your reference shelf beside your MT references. If you transcribe using Microsoft Word, get a *For Dummies* book on your version of Word, too. There's a good chance they'll come in handy.

Keeping Work in Its Place (And Interruptions Out)

Despite its many benefits, working from home is not as easy as most people anticipate. You'll have to train yourself, your family, your friends, and your neighbors regarding how this work-at-home stuff really operates. Boundaries that are automatic when you work at an "away" job can fall by the wayside. It's easy to get caught up in tasks that take you away from what actually earns you income, which is producing transcribed lines. The opposite can also occur; since your work is always nearby and you earn more by producing more, it's easy to slip into working incessantly, and who wants to do that?

These challenges are neither new nor insurmountable. Sticking to the following MT-tested guidelines can help you accomplish your work stuff during work hours:

- **Define a work schedule and stick to it 99 percent of the time.** That includes stopping on time, as well as starting on time. Work can expand to fill all available time if you let it; so can surfing the Internet and checking Facebook.

- **From the beginning, if someone asks you to do this or that during your scheduled work time, "since you're at home anyway," hitch up your spine and say no.** Inform her that you're working at that time and have to be at your desk. It may take a couple of repeats, but people will learn.

- **Eliminate distractions as much as possible.** If you want to work from home because you have young children, you'll still need someone to care for them during your work hours.

Home-work flexibility is a precious thing. If you want it to last, nurture and preserve it by creating a protective cocoon around your work time — and yourself. Check out Chapter 20 for additional tips on tending to yourself while attending to your work.

Chapter 19

Financial Considerations for Independent Contractors

· ·

In This Chapter

▶ Separating your business records from your personal records

▶ Setting up a business recordkeeping system

▶ Staying on the right side of Uncle Sam

▶ Protecting yourself and your stuff with insurance

· ·

*M*any companies that hire medical transcriptionists (MTs) want to hire them as independent contractors (ICs). In job listings, you'll see this indicated as "IC status." It means you and the hiring company are two businesses contracting with each other, instead of employer and employee. Here's what being an IC looks like for you and the hiring company:

✔ The hiring company doesn't have to pay employment taxes on your behalf. That becomes your responsibility.

✔ The hiring company doesn't have to provide and administer benefits or handle employee-related matters. It just cuts you a check and moves on.

✔ The hiring company can specify what you do (like produce *x* lines per week or turn around reports within 24 hours), but it can't control how you do it (for example, the hours you work or where you work from).

If you take a job as an IC, you're doing nothing less than deciding to launch your own business. You'll still have to work to get paid, but you'll have a lot more control over the *when, how,* and *for whom.* You'll also be responsible for stuff you may never have managed before, such as self-employment tax. Being in charge of your own work life is a thrilling proposition. It also can be a little scary. Welcome to self-employment!

In this chapter, you explore the financial keys to making IC status work in your favor. You see how and why to set up a recordkeeping system from which all else financial will flow, and how to stay on Uncle Sam's good side when it comes to taxes. After you read this chapter, *net income* may be your new favorite term.

Truth and consequences: Financial facts about going independent

You may have heard that working as an IC is essentially trading income for flexibility: In exchange for gaining control of your schedule, you have to be willing to take a financial beating. That can happen, but it's not a given.

Here are some of the benefits of working as an IC:

✔ You have more control over your work schedule. You can leave in the middle of the afternoon to run errands or meet a friend for coffee. You can work late at night instead of 9 to 5 if you prefer.

✔ You can take tax deductions for business-related expenses, like your computer, a second phone line used just for business purposes, and more.

✔ You have more control over how much work you do and how much you earn. You don't have to work 40 hours a week if you don't want to. And if you want to work more than 40 hours a week and have the work coming in to keep you busy, nothing is stopping you!

✔ You may be able to get insurance companies to issue you a health insurance policy even if you have a preexisting condition (see "Getting Insured," later in this chapter).

On the other hand, here are some of the drawbacks of being an IC:

✔ You spend more time dealing with paperwork and managing tax matters than you do when you're an employee.

✔ You have to pay taxes that an employer would pay on your behalf.

✔ You may not have a steady income, and even if you have steady work with regular clients, you don't have the same sense of security that you do when you're employed (although, especially in a tough economy, employees' sense of job security may be false).

✔ You don't have access to benefits partially or wholly funded by your employer, such as health or disability insurance and paid time off. This may not matter to you very much if you have another source, such as your spouse's employer. Part-time time employees rarely receive these benefits anyway, and many smaller MT employers offer on minimal or no benefits to anyone.

Don't get too tied up in knots over the decision. If you go IC and you don't like the results, you can always switch to an employee position later.

So, what's the difference between an independent contractor, a freelancer, and a sole proprietor? An *independent contractor* is a person or business that provides services to other businesses. *Freelancer* is just another name for independent contractor. And *sole proprietorship* is a term used on income tax forms to refer to an unincorporated business owned and operated by one person; it can be operated under the owner's name or under an assumed name, such as Magnificent Medical Transcription. (*Fictitious business name* and *DBA* [short for doing business as] are just different ways of saying assumed name.) If you're working on your own as an MT (regardless of whether you have a business name) and you aren't an employee, you're an IC or freelancer, and if you don't incorporate your business, you're a sole proprietor, too.

Keeping Good Records

Recordkeeping isn't just important come tax time — it empowers you to make the best choices for you and your business. Good records help you pay your bills on time and serve as your financial memory. Need another reason? It also helps you cut your tax bill.

As an IC, you get to deduct business-related expenses from the money you pull in before you pay a penny in taxes, like this:

revenue – expenses = net income (what you pay taxes on)

Revenue is the sum total of all the payments you receive, whether from one client or a dozen. Expenses are the sweet spot where you get to deduct the cost of things that you needed to operate your business. It includes things like

- Part or all of your Internet connection cost
- That new ergonomic keyboard and the mileage you drove to go get it
- The price of the bookkeeping software you purchased to track business finances
- Fees you pay an accountant to prepare the business portion of your tax return
- The cost of your trip to the AHDI annual conference and expo
- Other business-related stuff

Your recordkeeping system needs to

- ✔ Delineate personal and business expenses
- ✔ Track the data you need for tax purposes
- ✔ Produce reports whenever you need them so you can see where you're headed and remember where you've been

It needs two parts:

- ✔ A tracking/reporting system
- ✔ Organized storage for the check stubs, receipts, and other documents that back up your numbers

Setting up a business bank account and credit card

A good recordkeeping system makes it easy for you to separate business and personal transactions. One of your first steps when you decide to become an IC should be to consider opening separate bank and credit card accounts that you use strictly for business expenses.

Your business credit card doesn't need to be a fancy platinum card that comes with an annual fee. And it doesn't have to be a card geared toward businesses. Any credit card will do.

You aren't legally required to have separate bank and credit card accounts, but using dedicated accounts has a lot going for it:

- ✔ Life is easier at tax time.
- ✔ You won't have to copy deposits and expenditures from your personal accounts to your business records.
- ✔ If you're going to use a business name (for example, Magnificent Medical Transcription), you'll need a bank account under that name anyway.

Using separate accounts does have a few drawbacks:

- ✔ You'll have multiple accounts to reconcile. Thanks to modern bookkeeping software though, reconciling can usually be accomplished with just a few clicks.

- ✔ Adding a separate bank account may bring extra bank fees. But if you shop around, you can find bank accounts with very few fees. A good place to start looking is with online banks like Ally (www.ally.com) and ING Direct (www.ingdirect.com).

- ✔ You'll have an additional bill to remember to pay on time.

- ✔ You'll have the extra step of transferring money from the business account to your personal account. If both accounts are at the same bank, though, you can do it online in a few seconds.

Business checking accounts tend to have higher fees. If you're doing business under your own name and not a business name, you can open a second personal checking account instead of a business checking account and save on fees.

Tracking your income and expenses

You don't need to run out and learn double-entry bookkeeping in order to manage your own business finances. It's not like you're going to hire employees, lay in supplies, and start building widgets and shipping them to China. More likely, you'll start out with one or two transcription clients. You may expand your client base from there or keep it just like that.

Although you could track your business income and expenses using a handwritten ledger and a shoebox, there are better ways to go about it. Table 19-1 lists them and summarizes the pros and cons of each.

Table 19-1	Bookkeeping Methods	
Method	*Pros*	*Cons*
Handwritten ledger or notebook	It works even when the power is out.	It's slow, inflexible, and went out with the Stone Age.
Computer spreadsheet	You probably already have a spreadsheet application (such as Microsoft Excel) on your computer. It does the math for you.	You'll have to set it up and enter formulas. Unless you're a whiz with spreadsheets, you won't get many useful reports out of it.
Personal finance software	It's inexpensive, and you already may be using it for personal finances. You can automatically download transactions from your bank and credit card accounts to the software.	It doesn't provide much in the way of invoicing and client tracking functions. It wasn't designed to keep track of clients and receivables.
Small business bookkeeping software	It works a lot like personal finance software but includes better invoicing, business reporting, client and cost tracking, and lots of helpful reports.	It's more expensive than personal finance software, and you may find all the features and options confusing at first.
A professional accountant/bookkeeper	You can focus on transcription and keeping your clients happy. Meanwhile, your paperwork and business finances are being managed by a pro.	You won't have intimate knowledge of your finances. There may be a lag between when things happen and when your bookkeeper enters them into the system. It's also the most expensive option.

Using bookkeeping software

If you're planning to start out with just a client or two, there's no need to run out and purchase industrial-strength bookkeeping software right off the bat. You just need something you can use to record income and expenses, keep track of who owes you what when, and stay on top of tax matters.

If you have time on your hands, you can cruise around the web searching out and test driving free financial software. If you'd rather not, go straight to your favorite software outlet and pick out a version of Quicken or QuickBooks — they're both made by Intuit and widely supported by banks and financial services. Plus, there are plenty of how-to books and people who can help you out if you end up getting stuck.

Here are some of the differences between them:

✔ **Quicken Home & Business:** Quicken is a personal financial management system. It's primarily used to track household finances and investments, but the Home & Business version adds the ability to generate invoices and automatically categorize expenses as business or personal.

✔ **QuickBooks:** Essentially the go-to software for small businesses, QuickBooks is slightly more intimidating than Quicken but feature rich. It's strictly business — no personal finance or investment tracking. Even the base package allows you to track multiple clients individually, track receivables, and create statements, which Quicken does not. More accountants and tax professionals know QuickBooks than Quicken. Come tax time, you can often just provide access to your QuickBooks data file, and they'll take it from there. You can upgrade from business basics to a full-blown payroll management, inventory tracking, Swiss Army knife of business accounting, if you ever need to do so.

As you've probably guessed, QuickBooks costs more than Quicken; however, many people consider it well worth the extra money. Of note, you can transfer your data from Quicken to QuickBooks, but not the other way around.

Remember: If you purchase software to manage your business finances, make sure to deduct it!

Unless the thought of managing your own income and expenses triggers an urge to run screaming down the street, a software package is usually the best bet.

Just because you do your own bookkeeping doesn't mean you have to prepare your own tax return. Hand over the reports from your bookkeeping system and let a tax-prep person have at it!

Keeping the paper trail

Your business recordkeeping is only as good as the paperwork that stands behind it. That's true whether it's the physical documents or electronic versions. Things to hang on to include

✔ Receipts, invoices, and account statements related to your business expenses

✔ Bank and credit card statements that include business-related items

✔ Payment stubs from checks you receive

✔ Contracts you sign with clients or service providers

✔ Copies of insurance policies and warranties

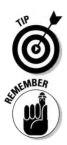

Look at Schedule C (available at `www.irs.gov/pub/irs-pdf/f1040sc.pdf`) to help you identify the types of things you should be recording.

If you receive electronic instead of paper statements, download them to your computer. Then back them up or print out and file them (or do both). Don't count on a financial institution to serve as your long-term document vault.

You'll also want to start a mileage log to record business-related driving. Those trips to the bank, post office, training seminar, or client's office are all potentially deductible. In 2012, the standard business mileage rate was 55.5 cents per mile. That may not sound like much, but over the course of a year, it can really add up. Your mileage log should include the date, destination, distance, and purpose of each trip. Make it easy on yourself: Store a pocket calendar in the glove box of your car or use a smartphone app — whatever's easiest for you.

You may have a lot of stuff to keep track of, but with minimal organization you can easily manage it. You really only need a few file folders. If you're the high-tech type, scan everything into your computer and use electronic folders.

How far you subdivide things is a matter of personal preference, but a basic set may include

✔ Business income

✔ Business expenses (invoices, receipts, statements, auto mileage)

✔ Home office deduction expenses (more on this later)

If you're planning to take the home office deduction, dedicate a folder to that rather than lumping it in with your general business expenses folder. It goes on a different form than your other business expenses, and keeping the supporting documents together makes things easier come tax time.

If you intend to hand the actual receipts over to an accountant (rather than reports from your bookkeeping software or the data file), organize your expenses into categories as you file them. Otherwise, you'll just have to do it later when it's harder to remember what they were for (or pay for the accountant to do it for you).

For simple all-in-one record storage, consider using an accordion-style folder. If you don't have the energy to label the sections yourself, pay a little more and get one that's already pre-labeled and divided for you. Each year, start a new one and store the old.

If you opt to scan your receipts and toss the originals, make sure you organize the scanned copies and make regular backups to an external device. If your hard drive heads south and takes your tax records with it, you'll need those backups.

Even if you're a compulsive cleaner, there are certain things you should never toss:

- ✔ Tax returns. (You can discard supporting materials like receipts and logs after seven years, but keep the actual returns forever.)

- ✔ Records pertaining to improvements you made to your home. (You'll need them when you sell it if you took the home-office deduction.)

- ✔ Insurance policies that are still in force.

- ✔ Warranties that haven't expired.

- ✔ Employment contracts.

Paying Uncle Sam

Going IC may do a lot of good things for you, but getting you out of paying taxes isn't one of them. When you work for yourself, you get to take some great tax write-offs. You also have to pay increased Social Security and Medicare taxes and manage paying them yourself. Most important:

- ✔ You have to make quarterly estimated tax payments. If you forget to do so, Uncle Sam can reach into your pockets and take out extra!

- ✔ As your own employer, you'll have to pay the portion of Social Security and Medicare taxes an employer pays on an employee's behalf. This is known as *self-employment tax.*

That's the major stuff. As long as you know about it and take care of it, it's really no big deal. It only becomes problematic if you don't do it. Two other notable things happen:

- ✔ Instead receiving a W-2 form at the end of the year, you'll receive one or more 1099 forms.

- ✔ Your federal income tax return will include additional forms.

Taxpayer ID numbers: What do you need?

You'll have to provide your client(s) with a taxpayer ID number (TIN) they can use for tax reporting. (They'll request your TIN on a W-9 form.) You have two options for TINs:

✔ **Social Security number (SSN):** Your SSN is a federal TIN used to identify an individual. It's a nine-digit number formatted like this: ###-##-####.

✔ **Employer identification number (EIN):** An EIN is a federal TIN used to identify a business entity. It's also a nine-digit number, but it's formatted like this: ##-#######.

If it's just you and no employees, you can use your SSN as your tax ID and you aren't required to get an EIN for your business. However, you may want one anyway. It's free, and it will keep your SSN private, because you can give clients your EIN instead. You can get one instantly by filling out the form on the IRS small business website: www.irs.gov/businesses/small.

Taxes are a complicated subject, and I can only touch on it here. If you want thorough information on preparing your taxes, check out *Taxes For Dummies* (Wiley). Also useful are *Working for Yourself: Law & Taxes for Independent Contractors, Freelancers & Consultants* and *Deduct It!: Lower Your Small Business Taxes,* both by Stephen Fishman, JD (Nolo).

Understanding self-employment tax

Self-employment tax is just another name for Social Security and Medicare contributions. If you had an employer, it would pay half and you would pay the other half. Because you're your employer, you have to pick up the whole tab. You figure self-employment tax by completing the Schedule SE form along with your annual federal tax return. It's calculated based on your net self-employment income, which, if you recall, means what's left after you deduct business expenses.

The standard self-employment tax rate is 15.3 percent (12.4 percent for Social Security and 2.9 percent for Medicare). If you're used to paying just the employee portion (7.65 percent), paying double can be a little stunning at first. But there's some good news: You get to deduct that extra half when calculating your adjusted gross income (AGI). AGI is the number used to determine your federal income tax. The lower it is, the lower your income tax bill will be.

Because of the 2010 Tax Relief Act, the self-employment tax rate was reduced to 13.3 percent (10.4 percent for Social Security and 2.9 percent for Medicare) for tax year 2011; Congress voted to extend the Tax Relief Act for tax year 2012 as well, but you can bet this extension won't last forever. For up-to-date information on the self-employment tax rate, go to http://tinyurl.com/38rac (this shortened URL will take you to the right page on the IRS website).

Making estimated tax payments

Income tax is a pay-as-you-go system. You pay in all year long, based on estimates of what your final tax bill will be. Then you have until April 15 to complete your annual tax return and calculate what you really owe. You either pay more or get some back.

When you're someone else's employee, your employer does the estimating and submits payments on your behalf. A portion is subtracted from your paychecks throughout the year as withholding and submitted to the public tax coffers. You don't get to get out of paying in all year long just because your income isn't coming from an employer. The difference is, you have to take over the task of estimating and making payments.

There are a couple of ways you can do it:

- ✔ Make quarterly estimated tax payments.
- ✔ Increase withholding from paychecks from an employer by enough to cover your self-employment income, too.

Estimated taxes are due four times a year (April 15, June 15, September 15, and January 15). Whoever you owe income taxes to (federal, state, and/or local) gets estimated tax payments. The mechanics of paying them is easy — just fill out the proper form and send it in with a check. Federally speaking, it's IRS Form 1040-ES. Whoever else you pay income tax to will have a corresponding form. You may expect them to be named similarly, but they're not. In New York State, it's form IT-2105. In North Carolina, it's NC-40. Go figure.

It is an approximation process, and the IRS doesn't expect you to get it smack on; however, it does expect you to come close. If you underpay, you can get hit with extra charges.

Estimated taxes payments made to municipalities are occasionally due on a different schedule. For example, in some cities, it's a once-a-year thing instead of quarterly.

If your income fluctuates, predicting this year's bill can get tricky. You can use a tax publication worksheet, tax prep software, an online calculator, or a tax professional to help you figure it out. As long as you pay estimated taxes equivalent to 100 percent of the previous year's tax bill or 90 percent of this year's bill, you'll be in the clear.

If you still have a "regular" job or file a joint return with someone who does, you can save yourself the hassle of submitting estimated tax payments by increasing the withholding from those paychecks.

Introducing 1099s

ICs receive 1099 forms instead of W-2s, so don't be surprised when they start arriving in the mail in January. The IRS gets copies, too. A 1099 form reports income paid to you during the year. Prior to 2011, the only 1099 you needed to know about was the 1099-MISC, but now there are two kinds an independent contractor may receive:

- ✔ **1099-MISC:** If a client pays you $600 or more over the year via check, direct deposit, or cash, you should receive a 1099-MISC from the client.

- ✔ **1099-K:** If the client pays you through a third party instead of directly, for example via a credit card or a payment system such as PayPal, it doesn't have to send you a 1099-MISC. You may instead receive a 1099-K from the payment processor, but only if certain transaction limits are surpassed. At the end of 2011, only payees who received over $20,000 *and* had over 200 credit/debit transactions were sent a 1099-K.

Sorting out 1099s is a much bigger headache for the people sending the forms than it is for the recipients. On your end, all you need to do is make sure that the numbers on any 1099 forms you receive match up with what you've already recorded in your records. There are two questions pretty much everyone who receives these forms asks about them:

- ✔ **Do I have to send 1099s in with my tax form?** No. Except in the extremely unusual case that the 1099 lists federal withholding *and* you're filing a paper return.

- ✔ **If I don't receive a 1099 from a client, do I still have to report and pay taxes on the income?** Yes! (You didn't think you'd get out of it because of a little missed paperwork did you?)

Tax information is always subject to change, so be sure to check up on it come tax time.

If you use tax prep software like TurboTax (www.turbotax.com) or H&R Block At Home (www.hrblock.com/tax-software), the software will do a lot of the legwork for you.

Adding a Schedule C to your tax return

Taxpayers who earn self-employment income report it on Schedule C, Profit or Loss from a Business. It's a two-page form. The first page contains the meat, including your bottom line: net profit. The second page contains additional sections that are only relevant to some situations. Here's how the form breaks down:

✔ **Part I: Income:** Business income you receive, before deducting anything, whether it's reported on a 1099 or not.

✔ **Part II: Expenses:** Business expenses except for those that fall under *business use of your home* (the official name for the home office deduction). Some categories of expenses are specifically listed, such as:

- Car and truck expenses (based on your mileage log)

- Legal and professional services (like accountant fees)

- Office expenses (office supplies and postage)

- Travel, meals, and entertainment expenses

- Contract labor (the amount you paid any ICs who did work for you)

- Other expenses (total amount of business expenses not specifically listed; you list them yourself in Part V of the form)

The fact that an expense isn't present as a line item on Schedule C doesn't mean that you aren't allowed to deduct it — it just means the IRS isn't reminding you to do so. That's what the "Other expenses" category is for — don't be afraid to use it!

The second page of Schedule C includes three additional sections:

✔ **Part III: Cost of Goods Sold:** You won't use this. It's only used by businesses that sell physical goods.

✔ **Part IV: Information on Your Vehicle:** Details about your vehicle use that support the "Car and truck expenses" you entered in Part II.

✔ **Part V: Other Expenses:** This where you itemize business expenses that the IRS isn't reminding you to deduct. The total carries to the "Other expenses" slot in Part I.

It's important to become familiar with Schedule C and stay up on the latest tax deductions related to self-employment. Read the instructions publication that accompanies Schedule C. You can get it at www.irs.gov/schedulec.

You also may end up completing additional forms to support specific deductions. To calculate the amount you can deduct for a home office, for example, you'll complete IRS Form 8829: Expenses for Business Use of Your Home (www.irs.gov/pub/irs-pdf/f8829.pdf).

Don't let talk about all these IRS forms intimidate you; any tax program or tax preparer can walk you through finding the right ones and filling them out. Go to the IRS website (www.irs.gov) for the latest forms and the tedious but crucial instructions that go with them. You also can call the IRS (800-TAX-FORM or 800-829-3676) and have forms and publications mailed to you for free.

Deducting everything you can

To pay as little in taxes as you legally can, you have to know about deductions that can lower your bill. This book can't give you specific tax advice, because, well, it just can't. You should always check with a tax advisor and not rely on advice from a book anyway. Some of the things you'll want to investigate include:

✔ **Home-office deduction:** The home-office deduction allows you to deduct a portion of the cost of maintaining your home or apartment from your taxable income. For example, if your qualifying home office takes up 10 percent of your home, you get to deduct 10 percent of your electricity bill, 10 percent of your rent, 10 percent of your insurance policy, plus additional items. If you're a homeowner, you can deduct even more (say, 10 percent of that new roof and 10 percent of real estate taxes). It can add up fast. IRS Publication 587: Business Use of Your Home (www.irs. gov/pub/irs-pdf/p587.pdf) lays out the rules and calculations.

Homeowners should be aware that taking the home-office deduction can have tax consequences years down the road. When you eventually sell your home you'll have to "recapture" part of what you deducted in previous years. The details go beyond the scope of this book, but essentially you may end up paying more taxes on profits from the sale of your home than you would have without the home-office deduction.

✔ **Self-employed health insurance deduction:** As of 2010, if you're self-employed, you can deduct the full cost of health insurance you purchase for yourself, your spouse, and/or your dependents. This only applies if you aren't eligible to participate in a health plan offered by an employer (yours or your spouse's). This is not a typo — it's true!

✔ **Retirement contributions:** Saving is rarely painless, but it can be a little easier when it comes with a tax deduction. As a self-employed person, you get to take advantage of particular types of tax-advantaged retirement savings accounts. They go by cryptic and clever acronyms, like SEP (rhymes with pep), IRA, and SIMPLE. See IRS Publication 560: Retirement Plans for Small Business (www.irs.gov/pub/irs-pdf/ p560.pdf) to pick the one that will best help you deposit and deduct.

The variety of deductions potentially available to you will likely change from year to year, so be thorough in your research.

Getting Insured

Being in business for yourself gives you additional things to protect, and it also gives you new ways to protect things you already have. It's a little-known secret that self-employment can be your gateway to health insurance you can't otherwise obtain. You also need to know what errors-and-omissions insurance is so you can decide whether to get it. And don't assume that your existing insurance covers all that stuff in your office against loss or damage — read the fine print.

Health insurance

Access to health insurance is a big concern for people considering life as an IC. Where will you get it? Can you get it at all? What if you have a preexisting condition and insurance companies won't issue you an individual policy? Healthcare reform legislation may make this a nonissue. In the meantime, there are multiple approaches you can take:

- ✔ If you have insurance coverage through an employer you're about to leave, you're probably eligible for COBRA.
- ✔ Purchase an individual health insurance policy.
- ✔ Obtain a group health insurance policy through your new business.
- ✔ Seek coverage through a state health insurance program.

COBRA

If your current employer has 20 or more employees, and you've been participating in the health plan for at least 180 days, you're most likely eligible for COBRA. It's a federally mandated program that lets you keep your current health plan for 18 months or longer by paying for it yourself. You can't be refused for any medical reason. Your current employer is in charge of setting this up for you. If you plan to go this route, don't wait long to get the ball rolling with your current employer — it's a limited-time opportunity.

Individual health insurance

If you're relatively healthy, an individual policy bought on the open market is another possibility. Plans are available in a variety of price ranges. You'll have to pass a health screening, and the insurer can decline to offer you a policy.

Small group health insurance via your newly formed business

In many states, if you qualify as a business, insurance companies can't deny you coverage. If you've ever been turned down based on a preexisting condition, this can be huge. The definition of *business* is not the same in every state. In some states, one legitimate employee (you) will do; in others, you'll need two or more. If you're fortunate enough to be in a state where a one-person business is eligible, your insurance agent may not even be aware of this option or offer it to you. The magic words to use are *company of one*. Then they'll know what you're talking about.

State insurance pools

Many states operate "risk pool" insurance plans that are open to people who can't get health coverage otherwise. You can find a list of them at www. naschip.org, which is the website of the National Association of State Comprehensive Health Insurance Plans (NASCHIP).

Errors-and-omissions insurance

A professional liability policy, also known as errors-and-omissions insurance, could save your bacon if someone sues you over a work matter. Stuff happens. Human beings make mistakes. And sometimes bad guys do things that cause our clients unexpected harm. For example, a computer virus may infect your system and spread to your client's, wiping out patient files. If the consequences are substantial enough, or if the client is angry enough, they may sue you.

In reality, people tend to sue entities with deep pockets, like corporations, not independent contractors and very small businesses. It's simple economics: There's not much point in suing Magnificent Medical Transcription if what you can potentially collect won't much more than cover your legal fees. However, it could happen. You may want to protect yourself with an errors-and-omissions policy, just in case. Even if you don't want such a policy yourself, you should know what errors-and-omissions insurance is, because the subject may come up in a discussion with a client. Now you know.

Homeowner's and renter's insurance riders

For many ICs, a basic homeowner's or renter's insurance policy is sufficient, but you should read your policy to be sure. You may want to add an in-home business rider to it. A rider is extra coverage for specific purpose that's added on top of a standard policy. You may want one because:

- ✔ **Your office equipment and furniture may not be insured as well as you think it is.** Don't assume your office computer, multifunction printer/fax/copy machine, high-end ergonomic chair, and the like are covered. Most residential insurance policies place a cap on coverage for office equipment and furniture. While you're at it, determine whether the policy provides replacement value or current value — you want replacement value.

- ✔ **A basic homeowner's policy doesn't cover business-related liability.** It may protect you if your neighbor trips on your stairs and develops a chronic back injury, but if a business client or vendor does the same, you'll likely be on your own. If clients never come to your home, you're probably in the clear on this one.

If you think you may need more coverage than your existing policy provides, call your insurance company and see what it has on offer. You may find you can gain substantial protection with just a little more money. Plus, the added cost is potentially tax deductible.

Insurance companies spend a lot of time figuring out what may happen to you and your stuff and how to sell you protection against it. You don't need to run out and buy every policy that includes the word *business*. For example, you may want disability insurance or business interruption coverage — or you may not. Talk to an insurance agent (or three). You don't have to do what they suggest, but it's wise to know what your options are.

The business hiring you doesn't get to designate you as an independent contractor for tax purposes but treat you like an employee. The IRS has very specific rules defining the difference between the two. If you're an IC, you're working for yourself and you aren't entitled to company-provided or govern-ment-mandated benefits, including unemployment and worker's compensation benefits. Some hiring firms may classify you as an IC, thus handing extra taxes and paperwork to you, yet still try to control you as if you're an employee. Whether they're doing it through ignorance or because they're trying to be sneaky, they don't get to have it both ways! When in doubt, send them to the IRS website to bone up on the difference. If they don't see the light, consider filing IRS Form SS-8: Determination of Worker Status for Purposes of Federal Employment Taxes and Income Tax Withholding (www.irs.gov/pub/irs-pdf/fss8.pdf), and the IRS will decide.

Chapter 20

Staying Healthy for the Long Haul

* *

In This Chapter

▶ Designing a workspace that will keep you healthy

▶ Avoiding carpal tunnel syndrome

▶ Combatting computer vision syndrome

▶ Stretching your way out of stuffed pretzel syndrome

▶ Preventing burnout from getting you in its grasp

* *

*T*he number one thing you can do to give your medical transcription (MT) career legs is take care of yourself physically and mentally — from the very beginning. The excitement of starting an interesting new career may have you blitzing through marathon keyboarding sessions and brushing aside such trivialities as a desk chair with a bad wheel, but that's exactly the kind of stuff that can bring it to an early end. Why risk it?

When you're keenly attuned to every syllable that comes over the headphones and every character on the computer screen, your muscles will tense up without your being aware of it. You'll realize it eventually — but probably not until you stand up hours later! Throw in a desk that's a bit tall, a chair that's a bit low, or a little glare on the computer screen, and it's a recipe for headaches, eyestrain, stiff muscles, and other forms of bodily revolt.

Fortunately, there's also a recipe to counteract the effects of protracted sitting. It has three main ingredients:

1. **Create a workspace that fits your body instead of forcing your body to fit an existing workspace.**

2. **Develop good, health-preserving habits.**

3. **Stick with them — even if you need to send yourself automated e-mail reminders or set an alarm clock to make it happen.**

Go Ergonomic or Go Home: Preventing Aches and Pains

Scientists have been studying how to make you comfortable (and, thus, healthy and productive) for years. It's called *ergonomics* — except when it's called *human factors engineering*. By any name, it's good news for people who spend a lot of time sitting in front of a computer, because it provides guidelines for setting up a workspace in a way that minimizes stress and strain on your body.

Your workstation: Assume the position

The goal of ergonomic workstation design is to facilitate a posture where your joints are naturally aligned in a neutral position. When sitting at your desk, that means:

- Hands, wrists, and forearms are aligned straight and roughly parallel to the floor.
- Shoulders are relaxed, with arms close in to the body and elbows bent 90 to 120 degrees.
- Thighs and hips are supported, with thighs parallel to the floor and knees at about the same height as hips.
- Feet should rest comfortably and well supported on the floor.
- Your back should have appropriate lumbar support, and your head should be balanced over your torso and level or bent slightly forward as you work.

Avoid arrangements that encourage you to lean forward, tilt your head back to look up at your monitor, reach to the side frequently to use a mouse or trackball, or prevent your feet from resting fully supported on the floor.

The guidelines of ergonomic design explain exactly how to set up your workspace to make all this happen. If your current equipment isn't very adjustable, try the workarounds suggested in Table 20-1, or buy new equipment that is.

Table 20-1	Troubleshooting Ergonomic Issues
The Problem	*The Fixes*
The desktop surface is too high.	Cut down the legs of the desk.
	Raise your chair height and use a footrest to effectively raise the floor height along with it.
	Use a keyboard drawer to lower the keyboard and mouse.
The desktop surface is too low.	Elevate the desk by placing concrete blocks or boards beneath the legs. Be sure whatever you use is strong and stable.
The computer monitor is too high.	Raise your chair height or lower your work surface.
The computer monitor is too low.	Elevate the monitor by placing books beneath it.
The computer monitor is too close due to lack of desk space.	Use a pull-out keyboard tray to create a deeper work surface.
The chair armrests are in the way.	Remove them or get a new chair.
The angle between your arms and your keyboard causes a slight upward or downward bending of your wrists.	Elevate the front or back edge of the keyboard to attain neutral wrist posture.
	Raise or lower your chair height or keyboard height.
When your chair is at the proper height to make everything else work, your feet are no longer resting comfortably on the floor, and your lower body alignment is thrown out of whack.	Use a foot rest to effectively raise the floor.

When you've achieved an ergonomically correct position, that doesn't mean you should sit in it as still as a statue. In fact, you should change positions whenever you feel the need. If you're leaning back a bit, sit up straight. Move your legs around beneath the desk. Stand up for a few minutes now and then. Avoid locking yourself in a single position to avoid tying your muscles in knots.

In the following sections, I cover the specifics on ergonomics for your workspace. There are a lot of details to keep in mind, but it's well worth the effort to match every one of them as closely as possible. Figure 20-1 shows how all these things work together.

Chapter 18 discusses technical specifications and features to look for when purchasing computer equipment.

Desk or other work surface (such as a table)

The work surface should be deep enough to allow you to place your computer monitor at least 20 inches from your eyes and straight in front of you. There should be plenty of room for you to place accessories such as your mouse and keyboard where you can easily reach them.

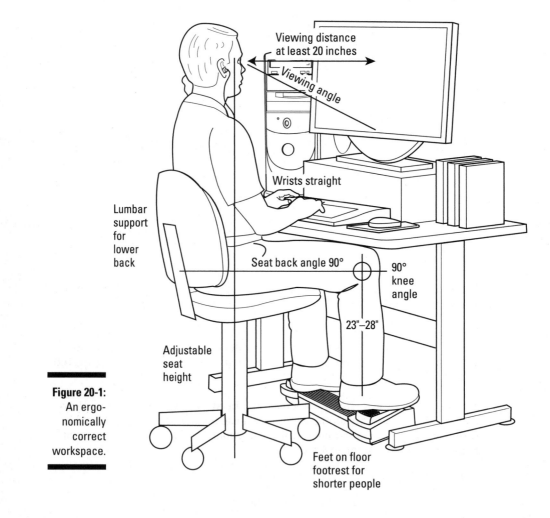

Viewing distance at least 20 inches

Viewing angle

Wrists straight

Lumbar support for lower back

Seat back angle 90°

90° knee angle

23"–28"

Adjustable seat height

Feet on floor footrest for shorter people

Figure 20-1: An ergonomically correct workspace.

The desk should provide adequate room for your legs to fit easily underneath and not be constricted. You should be able to reach your keyboard and mouse (or other pointing device) without hunching forward. Unless you're using a desk specifically designed for computer use, it may be necessary to add a keyboard drawer to accomplish this.

The all-important chair

Your chair absolutely must be adjustable. At the bare minimum, the chair height and back support should be adjustable.

The chair must provide adequate lumbar support, which means it fits the curve of your spine. Just because a chair provides lumbar support doesn't mean that support is in the right place for you, which is why it needs to be adjustable.

The seat should be comfortable and at angle that doesn't place pressure on the underside of your thighs when your feet are on the floor.

If the chair has armrests, they need to be adjustable, too, and soft. Ensure that they don't bump into your desk or otherwise prevent you from sitting the proper distance from your monitor and keyboard.

The chair should have a solid base with wheels so you can easily move into different positions. If your floor is carpeted, consider purchasing a plastic chair mat from an office supply store. It will allow you to move around more easily and protect your carpet from wear and tear.

Computer equipment

Although it won't hurt you to work from a laptop occasionally, it just won't suffice in the long run from an ergonomic perspective. If you're set on using one, connect it to a full-size keyboard and monitor.

Place your computer monitor directly in front of you, at least 20 inches way. The top of the screen should be at eye level or slightly below.

Keyboard height is very important. It should be at a level that allows you to keep your forearms approximately parallel to the floor and your wrists straight. A little low is better than a little high. You shouldn't have to stretch or hunch forward to reach the keyboard.

The mouse or other pointer device should be at the same level as your keyboard and immediately alongside it. If you use a keyboard tray, it should be wide enough to accommodate both the keyboard and the pointer device at approximately the same level.

The main computer system unit should be positioned so that it doesn't impede your movement and isn't at risk of being knocked over. On the floor beside the desk is a good option. Only put it under the desk if you still have plenty of leg room, though.

Your work environment

Once you're sitting pretty, the next step is to fine-tune work area lighting. Poor lighting can mess up your carefully obtained ergonomic position by causing your to tilt your head or angle your monitor differently in an attempt to see the screen better. Be especially vigilant for lighting that's excessively bright or glare on your computer screen; either one can trigger eye fatigue by making it more difficult to read. Position desk lamps so that they don't reflect light on the screen and limit brightness immediately around your monitor. As much as you may want to watch your attractive neighbor sunbathe, don't place your workstation so that you're facing a window. The sunlight coming from behind your monitor will bother your eyes in the long haul.

Over time, workspace ventilation can be an issue, too. If you're right beside or beneath an air vent, deflect the air so it doesn't blow directly on you, and don't point a fan directly on yourself. It may feel good at first, but most likely it will cause your eyes to become dry and uncomfortable.

The cornerstones to career longevity are using an ergonomically correct workstation and remembering to take frequent, short breaks.

Keeping Carpal Tunnel Syndrome at Bay

Because they spend so much time keyboarding, MTs are at risk of developing carpal tunnel syndrome (CTS), a painful and debilitating hand condition that results from a pinched nerve in the wrist. When caught early, the symptoms usually can be reversed, but if left untreated, permanent impairment can result. It's important to understand how CTS occurs so you can avoid it, or at least quickly recognize and react to any symptoms.

The carpal tunnel is a space between your wrist (carpal) bones and the major ligament that binds them together on the palm side of your wrist — right about where your wrists may rest on the edge of your desk or keyboard tray if you let them. The median nerve, which conveys signals back and forth to your hand, passes through it, along with a bunch of tendons that allow you to flex your fingers. If something causes the tunnel to narrow, most often swelling of the surrounding tissues, the median nerve can get compressed and CTS symptoms start. Typical symptoms include

✔ A vague aching in the wrist

✔ Tingling or numbness in your fingers or hand, especially the index, middle, and ring fingers

✔ Pain radiating to your hand and arm, especially on the palm side

The primary thing you can do to prevent CTS is to follow the ergonomic guidelines in this chapter, especially as they relate to keeping your wrists in line with your forearms. Don't rest your wrists on a hard surface such as the edge of your keyboard tray or desk. Give your hands and wrists frequent breaks by taking your fingers off the keyboard and gently stretching your hands and wrists. Try not to pound on the keys — just tap on them instead. Some transcriptions find that wearing light gloves that provide a bit of protection and wrist support helps prevent and alleviate symptoms, although it can be tricky to find gloves that do that without also impeding your typing ability.

If you start to develop CTS symptoms, that doesn't mean your MT career is doomed. Go see a healthcare provider, who will assess the severity of your CTS, probably recommend that you wear wrist splints at night, and help you determine how to proceed from there.

Dodging Computer Vision Syndrome

Staring at a computer monitor for hours on end can put a real strain on your eyes. Although there's no evidence that it causes long-term damage, it can certainly create significant short-term discomfort and impede your ability to work. Symptoms include dry eyes, blurred vision, difficulty focusing your eyes after a protracted period of looking at the monitor, light sensitivity, irritated, achy eyes, headache, and neck strain. These symptoms are all wrapped under the diagnostic umbrella called computer vision syndrome (CVS), although similar symptoms also occur in people in non-computer professions who do a lot of close-up work.

CVS is related to the way your eyes function when reading a computer screen. The nature of how computer letters are created on the screen makes them harder to read than letters printed on paper and forces the eyes to focus and refocus constantly. On top of that, people tend to blink a lot less often when concentrating intently on a computer screen, which leads to dry, irritated eyes.

To ward off the unpleasant symptoms of computer vision syndrome, experts suggest the following:

✔ Follow the 20-20-20 rule: Every 20 minutes, rest your eyes by looking away from the monitor and focusing on an object 20 feet away for 20 seconds.

✔ Avoid sitting where air is flowing past your face from a vent or fan, potentially drying your eyes.

✔ Follow ergonomic guidelines for proper lighting, because glare or overly bright lights can aggravate the problem.

✔ Make a conscious effort to blink. Over-the-counter artificial tears also can help alleviate dry-eye symptoms.

Avoiding Stuffed Pretzel Syndrome

If the only time you get up from your desk is for a trip to the restroom or to walk back and forth to the kitchen for a snack, you're at high risk for stuffed pretzel syndrome. The primary symptoms are muscle aches and weight gain. After hours sitting at your desk, your muscles will feel stiff, tired, and tied in knots like a pretzel when you finally stand up. You're also likely to be less active overall, because all that immobility leads to aches and pains and, as counterintuitive as it sounds, fatigue. The stuffed part of the syndrome, of course, results from the combination of inactivity and too many trips to the kitchen.

Avoiding stuffed pretzel syndrome is easy: Get up regularly to stretch or move around a bit (to somewhere other than the kitchen), and keep a variety of low-calorie, healthy snacks and beverages in the kitchen that you can grab when you do end up there.

Sitting down used to be what people did to take a break from hard work, but now we know it's important to take a break from the hard work of sitting!

Beating Burnout

Virtually everyone goes through patches of job stress and comes out fine on the other side, but when the rough patch seems to never end, you may have run head-on into burnout. Work-at-home MTs are especially at risk for it. When your desk is just a few steps away and you're paid based on production, that desk can pull at you like a magnet. Before you know it, you can end up living to work instead of working to live. Add in a liberal dollop of isolation and an employer who keeps demanding more and more from you, and you easily can end up constantly stressed out and overwhelmed.

As with most unpleasant conditions, it's best to avoid it in the first place, but even if burnout is already starting to wrap its tentacles around you, it's not too late to deploy a counteroffensive. The following strategies can help keep burnout away or send it packing:

✓ **Set limits and stick to them.** Work will expand to fill all available time if you let it. Determine how much you're willing (and realistically able) to work, and set specific work hours accordingly. You can go back to being more flexible later if you want to. Don't be afraid to say no to unreasonable work demands. A request to work extra now and then is reasonable; demanding it constantly is not. If you quit today, your employer would find a way to get the work done without you, so don't even entertain feelings of guilt about not agreeing to every request for more of your time.

✓ **Remember that you always have choices.** You're not locked into your current employer, your current work schedule, or even working as an MT. There are always alternatives, even if they aren't immediately appealing. You can change employers, change hours, even change to a new career if it really comes down to it. Just recognizing that you do have options can loosen the grip of stress considerably. It also can help you take a fresh look at your current situation and realize that although you've encountered a rough spot, with perhaps a few adjustments, a return to smooth sailing awaits on the other side. Choose to live sustainably.

Part V
The Part of Tens

The 5th Wave   By Rich Tennant

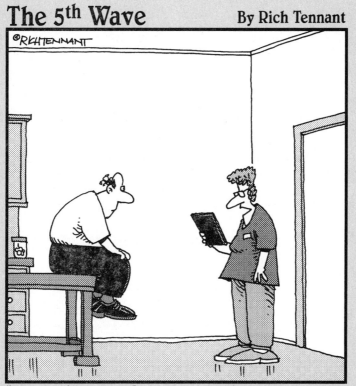

"Sorry I'm late, Mr. Peters. We're still working out the kinks in our new medical transcription speech recognition software. Now, let's take a look at that high bug pressure of yours."

In this part . . .

Good things come in tens, especially in this section. You'll discover ten factors that contribute to career success, bust ten myths about medical transcription, and get a lead on ten awesome online resources you'll probably want to bookmark.

Chapter 21

Ten Keys to Career Success

In This Chapter

▶ Starting out strong

▶ Building a lasting and satisfying career

Desire and determination underlie every successful medical transcription (MT) career, but it doesn't hurt to have a few guiding principles handy too. This chapter provides ten of them to help you build a satisfying and enduring career.

Use the Right Tools

You wouldn't try to mow a lawn with a pair of scissors. If you try to transcribe on a laptop at the dining room table with the Internet as your only reference, you're pretty much attempting the same thing. You can equip yourself with the tools of the trade without breaking the bank. A solid reference library and a well set-up work area aren't "nice to have" — they're required. The investment you make in them will pay off many times over.

Your MT tools don't have to be shiny, new, and top of the line, but they do need to be present and functional. You need a space where you can work undisturbed on a work surface that isn't being used for anything else. It can be a desk you pick up at a yard sale or the latest whiz-bang adjustable workstation with 32 settings. As far as the computer, some employers will ship one to your door loaded and ready to go; all you have to do is plug it in and turn it on. If you need to provide your own, which is not uncommon, there's no need to go for a high-end model unless you want to. Performing medical transcription doesn't require a lot of computing power. You can easily get along with a budget-priced or older computer, just as long as you can set it up in an ergonomically correct manner. For help with computer specs, turn to Chapter 18.

As for your starter reference library, if your budget is tight or you just enjoy being frugal, pick up as much as you can used from sources like Amazon. com and eBay. If you go this route, be mindful of which versions and editions you're purchasing. A drug reference such as the *Quick Look Drug Book* (Lippincott Williams & Wilkins) needs to be the latest version available. A medical dictionary, such as Stedman's (www.stedmans.com) or Dorland's (www.dorlands.com), doesn't have to be up to the minute to be incredibly useful, as long as it's recent. The same is true of general word and phrase books. If you'll be doing any acute-care transcription, it's worth springing for the latest edition of a medical and surgical equipment words book, because new equipment and devices hit the market every day.

Craft a Regular Work Routine and Stick to It

The familiar saying, "Failing to plan is planning to fail," is right on the mark for home-based MTs. Determine what your work schedule needs to be, and adhere to it just as if you were going to an office each day. If you're employment arrangement allows it, pick a structure and work hours that leverage your personal strengths. If you're most productive first thing in the morning, start work at the crack of dawn. If you're a night owl, schedule yourself to hit the keyboard when others are hitting the sack. If you don't want to or can't complete your work in a single sitting, divide your workday hours into two sessions with a break in the middle.

Whatever schedule you come up with, stick to it. This can require major self-discipline but brings multiple payoffs. First, it immeasurably increases the likelihood you'll get the work done. When someone wants to drop by for a bit of coffee and conversation, it's very easy to reply, "I'm sorry, but I'm working until 7 today. How about tomorrow?" Working a set schedule also triggers the power of habit. Your brain will come to know that certain times of day are dedicated to transcription work and will be primed to swing into gear when those times arrive. There still will be days when only willpower will get you to your desk, but once you're there, the power of habit will swing into action.

Become a Master of Faster

Love it or hate it, medical transcription is a pay-for-production proposition. You have to be quick and efficient to earn a living in this profession. To crack the upper echelons of MT income, you'll need to be faster still, without sacrificing accuracy. This isn't just a matter of increasing your keyboarding speed, although that matters; it's about employing proven techniques to elevate your production far above the simply fast fingered.

Many MTs have a grip on the basics, but becoming a true speed demon requires, paradoxically, more time. Who has time to memorize a lot of keyboard shortcuts, reorganize surroundings for efficiency, and study systems created and honed by superstar MTs? You do, if you choose to. Chapters 8 and 9 can help.

Mind Your Body

Take ergonomics seriously from day one; don't wait until you start getting aches and pains from spending long hours at a desk. Although you can get away with ignoring ergonomics for a while, it will catch up with you. At the very least, you'll end up uncomfortable, but that can progress to a debilitating condition such as carpal tunnel syndrome that could put your MT career on hold or end it entirely. Chapter 20 provides detailed advice about setting up an ergonomically correct workstation, along with additional steps to help you continue to working comfortably for a long time to come.

Project Professionalism

Don't let a casual work environment trigger a casual attitude. Whether you're wearing your pajamas and slippers or dressed to impress, be sure to don the hat of professionalism every day. As a remote worker, how you look is irrelevant, but how you come across in e-mail and phone calls becomes more important than ever. You don't have to turn yourself into Fannie Formal, but there are several things to keep in mind to ensure you come across as professional:

✔ Take the extra minute to proofread work-related e-mails for grammar and clarity before hitting send. Remember that the reader can't see your facial expressions or hear the tone of your voice, which creates great potential for misinterpretation. Reserve the clever smileys for personal communications.

✔ Don't attempt to multitask by continuing to type or tossing in a load of laundry while on the phone with an employer or client. They'll hear you, and they'll feel disrespected.

✔ Receive criticism gracefully. Keep your cool and respond appropriately, even it strikes you as patently unfair. Make this your mantra: When you feel compelled to act, hesitate first.

Above all, be dependable and responsible, and always deliver work that you can take pride in.

Get a Mentor

Support and advice from a trusted advisor is valuable in any profession. For medical transcriptionists who work independently, it's a major leg up. Seek out an experienced MT who is willing to answer your questions and provide support and guidance.

The best way to find a mentor is to ask other MTs you know and respect if they would be willing to serve as a mentor or can suggest a colleague. If you don't know any working MTs yet, seek out earlier graduates from the program you attended. Message boards operated by the MT program you graduated from can be an ideal place to look. If you're still mentor-less, scout for candidates on MT community websites. Prowl the message boards for contributors who display a positive attitude and have been contributing to the community for at least a year and working as MTs longer than that.

Don't expect a mentor to answer e-mails immediately or tell you exactly what to do. A mentor's role is to advise, guide, and provide support and encouragement. What you do with that advice and whether you follow the guidance is entirely your responsibility.

Above all, be sure to show your appreciation to anyone who takes the time to mentor you. When you get some experience under your belt, you can return the favor by mentoring other fledgling MTs.

The AHDI Annual Conference and Expo (ACE) is an ideal place to meet other MTs, interact with prospective employers, and potentially find your mentor. For the date and location of the next one, visit the AHDI website (www.ahdi online.org).

Tune In to the MT Network

When you're sitting at your desk by yourself and the only sounds are the voice of a distant dictator and the tick of the ceiling fan, remember this: You are not alone. Working from home can be fantastically freeing, but at times it may leave you feeling isolated. If there is no co-worker beside you, who do you turn to for opinions on professional issues? How do you stay attuned to what's happening in your field? The answer to both questions is to join the vibrant online community of home-based MTs. You'll be able to meet other MTs, learn about new references and resources, and keep abreast of industry news such as which companies are acquiring, hiring, or laying off. It's not, however, a good place to vent frustrations (more on this later), an activity best reserved for conversations with a few close friends.

Your supervisor, co-workers, and other MTs you know will most likely be happy to share their favorite virtual MT watering holes. MTDaily (`www.mtdaily.com`) and MT Gab (`www.mtgab.com/forum`) are great places to connect with other home-based MTs.

Critical to benefitting from the MT network is to tune in periodically, not constantly. If you find yourself visiting message boards to the point where it begins to interfere with your productivity, relegate check-in time to a particular slot in your schedule. The online MT community is very welcoming and can easily slide from support source to distraction in no time.

Keep Your Balance

Most people view their work schedules from the perspective of when they'll work, not when they won't. It's more beneficial to instead look at it as both a framework to ensure you work and a container to keep work in its place. With your office just a few steps away and the potential to earn more if you work more, that desk can pull on you like a magnet. If you're not careful, one day you may wake up and realize you're spending a lot more time there than you ever intended, and the rest of your life is paying the price.

The first thing to go is usually personal time — when you would have gone to the gym, caught lunch with a friend, or watched the evening news. Then the squeeze extends to family time, which threatens to become a burden instead of a pleasure. Work will expand to fill all available time if you let it, and more. You won't be happy, your family won't be happy, and physical and mental burnout are likely imminent.

So, how do you resist the magnetic pull of your desk? Give equal power to the other magnets in your life: your sense of personal well-being, your family and friends, causes you care about — all the non-work elements of your life. Build a life schedule, not just a work schedule. Make short-term goals, but maintain a long-term perspective. Don't expect work and not-work to stay neatly in their slots all the time, but if one begins to blot out the other, back away, rebalance, and start again.

Don't Get Sucked into a Negativity Vortex

This one is so important that you should write it on a sticky note right now and fasten it to your computer monitor or somewhere else you'll see it every day.

It's human nature to get frustrated with your job from time to time, no matter what it is. It's also human nature to seek out confirmation and support when that happens. But what do you do if you work from home and there's no one around to discuss it with? A lot of people go to an online MT community and air their grievances there. People who are happy and doing well rarely go online and post about it, but for someone who is frustrated, discouraged, or lonely, the opportunity to complain publicly yet anonymously can be enormously attractive. As a result, negative opinions and events appear much more prevalent than they actually are.

You can see this principle in action in any online community, including MT gathering spots. At some of them, the message boards are rife with griping about the medical transcription field: The pay is too low, the work is thankless, the dictators are too difficult. Look a little more closely, and you may discover that the same people have been doing the complaining for years! Obviously, they feel the benefits outweigh the drawbacks, or they would've found another job long ago — but drawbacks are more interesting to post about.

Griping tends to attract more griping. A complaint posted to a message board can remain visible for years, just waiting for someone who's having a bad day or feeling bored to come along and add to it. It can become a perpetual mass of negativity that beckons all to join in. Even on a bad day, resist the temptation. When you've tumbled into the vortex of negativity, it's very difficult to extricate yourself.

Be Adaptable, Embrace Change, Nourish Your Career

MTs must continuously learn new terminology, new technologies, and new ways of working, something that most accomplish with pleasure and no small amount of pride. That's always been true, but the pace of technological change has picked up considerably in recent years, and the changes are coming larger and faster. It's exciting and scary at the same time. You can hold your breath, squeeze your eyes closed, and wait for this wave of change to crash over you, or you can catch a thrilling ride on it.

If you're going to surf instead of sink, start by sizing up the incoming wave and the angles you might take. Right now, that means keeping a close eye on the migration to electronic health records (EHR) and changes to healthcare documentation regulations, and envisioning your place within them.

The incoming wave of EHR is powered by the interaction of three systems: healthcare, information technology (IT), and government. Healthcare providers generate the information that goes into the EHR; information technology experts supply the know-how to collect, digitize and manipulate it; and legislative experts pass laws to govern privacy and protection of the data (see Figure 21-1). There's a place at the center of this triangle for experts who get the big picture and are intimately familiar with the desired end result: a clear, accurate, understandable medical record that conforms to legal protections and facilitates the delivery of safe and effective patient care. These experts will keep abreast of health information regulations, grasp the big picture of how the technology works, and remain fluent in the language of medicine. It's a role tailor-made for medical transcriptionists.

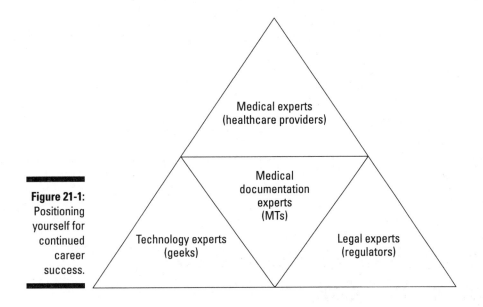

Figure 21-1:
Positioning yourself for continued career success.

EHR is the wave of change MTs face today, but future opportunities may arrive in an entirely different form. Do the things successful MTs have always done — learn new terminology, new technologies, and new ways of working — and you'll always have the chance to ride high on the incoming surf. Look to the horizon with anticipation, and pick your angle.

Chapter 22

Ten Myths about Medical Transcription

. . . .

In This Chapter

▶ Getting the true story about medical transcription

▶ Telling the difference between fact and fiction

. . . .

There's a lot of misinformation floating around about the ins and outs of a medical transcription career. Some of it comes from honest misconceptions; the rest comes from training companies that want your money. Medical transcription (MT) is interesting and challenging. You can train from home and work from practically anywhere you can get an Internet connection. There are opportunities to work nontraditional hours, part-time or full-time, as an employee or as self-employed independent contractor. MT has a lot going for it. It isn't, however, a free ticket to prosperity with no strings attached.

In this chapter, I outline the most common myths about medical transcription. Too many people throw away money on bad courses or invest a lot of time and money to launch an MT career only to discover it's not what they expected. It's easy to make mistakes if you have no way to know fact from fiction. This chapter gives you a way.

You'll Make $50,000 a Year Working from Home

This particularly alluring myth frequently appears in advertisements promising to take you from zero to MT in a matter of months — just come to our free seminar to find out how! Don't believe it, and don't sign up for training (or even attend a seminar) from any company that makes such a claim. Are there MTs who make $50,000 a year? Yes, but they're few and far between. A quick trip to the U.S. Bureau of Labor Statistics (BLS) website reveals that the average annual salary for a full-time MT is closer to $34,000. You're probably planning to be above average (aren't we all?) but it'll take you a while to get there. In addition, many MTs work part-time, so be sure to factor that into your earnings calculations. Chapter 3 is chock-full of additional facts on MT pay and employment options you'll want to know.

You Can Work and Take Care of the Kids at the Same Time

If you're picturing yourself tapping away at the keyboard while your little darling plays quietly at your feet, pinch yourself and wake up! There's no way you can transcribe medical reports and take care of children at the same time. MT work requires intense concentration and undivided attention, two things that aren't compatible with supervising little ones (or much of anything else). If you have young children at home, you'll need to arrange for childcare during your work hours or work while they're sleeping. MT is a job that has more flexibility than most, but it's hard work that requires your undivided attention. By the way, not all MTs work from home; some work on-site, and others split their time between a home office and an on-site office.

If You Can Type Really Fast, You're in Like Flynn

The ability to type at warp speed is a great asset, but it isn't an automatic ticket to success as an MT. The things that really make the difference are largely mental:

- An inquisitive mind and love of language so you can learn (and keep learning) all those medical terms
- An independent, pressure-resistant mindset
- The ability and motivation to concentrate intently for extended periods of time

If you have these traits plus determination, chances are, you can learn the practical skills you'll need, including how to type fast.

You, Too, Can Become an MT with Little or No Training

Unless you have formal medical transcription training, your résumé will never make it into the "to interview" stack. The training must be from a recognized, reputable source, such as a community college program or well-established medical transcription school. Otherwise, you're toast. Your cousin Joe Bob might know someone who knows someone whose sister became a medical transcriptionist without formal education, but that was probably back in the days when car bumpers were still made of metal.

Plan on spending a bare minimum of nine months preparing for your new career. You'll study anatomy and physiology, medical terminology, formatting of the different report types, and many more skills you may not anticipate needing but definitely will. When you graduate, you'll have that crucial formal training to include on your résumé and the know-how to do the job.

Speech Recognition Technology Will Make Medical Transcriptionists Obsolete

Speech recognition technology (SRT) is in widespread use as a way (in theory) for medical facilities to cut transcription costs. Working MTs refer to it as "speech wreck," because the results sometimes have more in common with a multicar pileup than a quality healthcare document. Under ideal dictation conditions, SRT can do a decent job, but it takes very little to send things awry.

An increasing number of MTs are finding their job descriptions have expanded to include speech recognition editing (finding and fixing the speech wrecks). As amazing as it is, SRT just isn't up to the task of producing quality reports despite thick accents, background noise, bungled grammar, words that sound identical but mean different things, and other concerns that MTs routinely handle. Nor is a computer program likely to notice if a distracted physician dictates information in the wrong section of a report or suddenly starts saying "right kidney" instead of "left kidney."

Despite its substantial shortcomings, SRT seems to be here to stay. Because the results of SRT are unreliable and require constant supervision, it now figures into what MTs do on a daily basis. Speech recognition has added a fresh twist to the ever-evolving MT profession, not made it obsolete.

Electronic Health Records Will Eliminate the Need for Medical Transcriptionists

This is only true in the minds and marketing materials of people who sell EHR software. Somewhere along the way, the idea of digitizing medical information seems to have become equated with transforming the recording of healthcare details into an entirely point-and-click process, but it's increasingly evident that it can't be done.

Some elements of healthcare documentation are enhanced by restricting input via check boxes and drop-down lists, but for some things, fill in the blanks just doesn't cut it. Healthcare providers need a way to incorporate narrative observations, opinions, and conclusions — in other words, dictation. The move to electronic health records is nothing less than a seismic shift in the healthcare documentation process, but MTs continue to be needed to help make EHR work.

Most Medical Transcription Work is Being Outsourced Overseas

Everything else seems to be going to cheaper, offshore workforces — why not medical transcription? After all, who can afford to pass up a chance to save some green? Medical transcription began going abroad in the 1990s, and more was headed that way, but then things changed. In 2010, changes in federal laws related to protecting patient health information made compliance with federal Health Insurance Portability and Accountability Act (HIPAA) rules an even higher priority for medical transcription companies and healthcare facilities. In order to achieve tighter control over patient information, it's being kept closer to home. As a result, less medical transcription is going overseas. Many of the organizations that were piloting offshore transcription have terminated those flight plans and are keeping it squarely inside U.S. borders.

Getting Certified Is the Best Way to Break Into Medical Transcription

Any advertisement that entices you to "become a certified medical transcriptionist" is feeding you a line of hogwash. You don't need a certification or a license to become an MT. There is a Certified Medical Transcriptionist (CMT) credential, but it's not an entry-level kind of thing, and no training program can give it to you. You may opt to earn it eventually, but you'll need at least two years of experience under your belt first. Even then, you'll have to pass a rigorous exam that will test your medical knowledge and transcription skills across multiple medical specialties.

There's a second MT credential program that is open to new graduates and entry-level MTs, but it's not particularly sought after by employers and certainly not required. The Registered Medical Transcriptionist (RMT) program is operated by the Association for Healthcare Documentation Integrity (AHDI), the same professional organization that created and manages the CMT. Nobody can award you this one either; the only way to get it is to pass the RMT exam.

If you feel like challenging yourself or want to add a little extra zip to your résumé, you may elect to earn it, but it's strictly optional. You'll need formal training to break into medical transcription, but not certification. Chapter 4 explains the must-haves and nice-to-haves for breaking in to the MT field.

It's Low-Stress Work

You may think medical transcription is a low-pressure job. How hard can it be to listen to what somebody says and type it up in a report? A lot harder than you can ever imagine until you've actually done it. You'll be astounded by what comes across your headphones — guaranteed!

For starters, medical dictation often arrives amply stocked with background noise and interruptions — and don't forget the crackers (dictators seem to frequently have a mouthful of them). It includes words you haven't ever heard before and have no idea how to spell, especially at first. Many times, a thick foreign accent will be slathered on top. So, let's just say the clarity isn't always the best. . . .

Even in the unlikely event that you have dreamy dictators in an ideal dictation environment, you're still not home free. There's still productivity pressure — it looms over everything else. Your paycheck will be tightly linked to how many reports you transcribe, how quickly, and how perfectly. High quantity and high quality don't always go hand in hand, but it's part of your job to make them do so. The amount of productivity pressure you face will be affected by the type of work you do, how much you enjoy it, and how good you are at it. In any event, very few MTs would describe their work as low-stress.

Real Men Don't Become Medical Transcriptionists

Okay, maybe nobody says that, but you may get that impression when researching the field. The current crop of MTs is overwhelmingly female, but men and women are equally capable of becoming excellent MTs. It's not any harder for a man to break into the field than it is for a woman. As more men seek out work they can do from home or on a flexible schedule, they're discovering medical transcription. MT employers care how many reports you can produce, how fast, and how accurately. Whether you're female or male, old or young, a marathoner or wheelchair-bound doesn't matter. Real men can — and do — become medical transcriptionists.

Chapter 23

Ten Great Online Resources

In This Chapter

▶ Knowing where to turn for more information

▶ Zeroing in on top websites for medical transcriptionists

*T*he ten websites in this chapter won't enhance your love life, ensure eternal youth, or snag you a million-dollar check from Nigeria, but they're incredibly useful nonetheless. Whether you want to hob-knob with other medical transcriptionists (MTs), spell the name of a doctor who has more vowels in his name than patients in his office, or figure out what you can deduct on your Schedule C, there's a site for that. You'll find ten of the most useful right here.

Meet at the Corner on Facebook

The Medical Transcription Networking Corner Group on Facebook (www.facebook.com/groups/MTCorner) is a fast-growing online community of MTs, both knowledgeable and new. The attitude here is particularly positive, and if you post a question, you'll start receiving answers almost instantly. It's a great place to seek advice, swap strange but true dictation tales, and socialize with fellow MTs. You know you needed another excuse to get on Facebook. Here it is!

Check Multiple Sources with OneLook

This specialized search engine allows you to search multiple dictionaries with one click. Use OneLook (www.onelook.com) to quickly look up medical words and phrases, acronyms, and abbreviations. OneLook's true beauty lies in the amazing advanced search that goes far beyond what other lookup sites offer. Take a few minutes to review the wildcard examples, and you'll be power searching in no time. You also can customize the result contents and appearance, and OneLook will remember them the next time you visit.

Find What's-Her-Name from Somewhere

HealthGrades (www.healthgrades.com) is a tool for connecting consumers with healthcare providers; it also happens to be a great way for an MT to connect with the correct spelling of an unfamiliar physician name or hospital. You can search by location, provider name, and specialty. The best matches will start popping up before you finish entering in your query.

Solve Drug Problems

When you need to figure out an unclear drug name or dosage, there's a good chance Drugs.com (www.drugs.com) can help. It includes information on more than 24,000 prescription drugs, over-the-counter medicines, and supplements. You can search by drug name or dosage details, or even get a list of drugs used to treat a particular condition.

The phonetic and wildcard searches are ideal for MT needs. If you can take a half-decent guess at a drug name, you can use either one to help pin it down. Even the standard search will inquire "Did you mean Motrin?" if you enter "mitrin," but if you switch to the phonetic search, an extended list of possibilities will pop up, including Motrin, Midrin, and Materna.

When using search tools to pin down medical terms or drug names, be extremely alert for sound-alike matches. For example, Motrin and Midrin are distinct drugs, and either one might be used to treat headaches. Nor would you want to mix up peroneum and perineum, which are wildly different body parts. If your research doesn't leave you absolutely certain what the dictator actually said, don't guess!

Samplify Your Work Life

Need more samples? Stedman's knows you do, and Stedmans@Work (www.stedmans.com/atwork) is the doorway to a repository that includes more than 400 transcribed reports. Whether you need help deciphering an acupuncture office note or a detailed surgical procedure (rhinoplasty, anyone?), this is a good place to look. The collection is searchable by keyword, specialty, and report type. You can even download the samples to your own computer, if you want. Stedman's print and electronic medical references are among the most widely used by MTs, and this page also serves as a jumping-off point to Stedman's product catalog.

Talk Productively about Productivity

The Productivity Talk (www.productivitytalk.com) forum is an ideal place to get and give tips and share resources for making the most of software-productivity boosters. Everyone who wants to master computing shortcuts is welcome, and many efficiency-minded MTs participate. If you have a question about a particular word-expander program, such as Instant Text or Shortcut, someone here will know the answer. You'll also find a pile of keyboard shortcuts and Microsoft Word macros, along with advice on integrating all these goodies with specific medical transcription platforms.

This is also the perfect place to explore and discuss the merits of different shortcut systems. It also presents an opportunity to swap word expander dictionaries with other MTs instead of creating your own from scratch, one of the biggest time-savers of all.

If you're not sure what word expanders and shortcut systems are, head over to Chapter 9 right now!

Get Industrial-Strength Updates

Regardless of whether you choose to become a member of the Association for Healthcare Documentation Integrity (AHDI), the AHDI website (www.ahdionline.org) is worth checking out regularly. You'll find information on the Annual Conference and Expo (ACE), which is a great opportunity to meet other MTs and potential employers, hone your current skills, and develop new ones. This is also the place to sign up for Registered Medical Transcriptionist (RMT) and Certified Medical Transcriptionist (CMT) professional exams. AHDI also posts articles about industry trends and "best practices" guidelines.

Go Shopping for Transcription Gear

Sooner or later you're going to want some new stuff. It may be better headphones, a pair of comfort typing gloves, or a foot pedal to replace the one your dog mistook for a chew toy. There's more than one place you can get such wondrous treasures, but TranscriptionGear.com (www.transcriptiongear.com) is among the best. It has been around a long time, provides excellent customer service, and even has a clearance rack.

Healthy Computing in Exquisite Detail

Healthy Computing (www.healthycomputing.com) has everything you could possibly want to know about office ergonomics and then some. It offers detailed tips and photos for setting up every aspect of your workspace and buyer's guides for choosing ergonomically friendly everything, from keyboards to telephones.

If you already have aches and pains, go to the "Your Health" section, select "Causes of Discomfort," and then select the body part that hurts — you can identify ergonomic issues that could be triggering your pain.

If you take your work on the road, be sure to visit the "Mobile Ergonomics" section.

Tax Advice Straight from the IRS

The IRS Self-Employed Individuals Tax Center (www.irs.gov/businesses/small/selfemployed) is a must-visit if you're working as an independent contractor or considering doing so. You'll find explanations (in plain English, believe it or not!) about federal tax facts that apply to you. It includes

✔ How to calculate and pay federal estimated taxes, including self-employment tax

✔ How to file your annual federal tax return and which forms to use

✔ Information about tax deductions that may apply to you

✔ Downloadable versions of all tax forms and instructions

There's also a very helpful interactive Small Business/Self-Employed Small Business Tax Workshop. Tax topics are broken out into individual lessons, so you can skip the boring stuff that doesn't apply to you. You also can skip out in the middle of a lesson and pick up where you left off later.

Be sure to visit the websites for your state and municipality, too. To help you find them quickly the IRS maintains a state-by-state list of links at http://tinyurl.com/j6t71.

Part VI
Appendixes

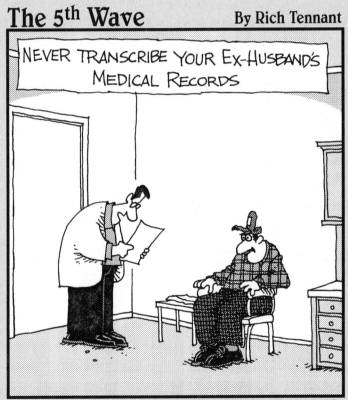

"Let's see, you're my 46-year-old dirtbag with acute cheapskateitis?"

In this part . . .

*I*t's impossible to have too many examples when starting out, and you'll find a helpful collection of them here. If transcription-related jargon has you baffled, dip into the glossary in Appendix A. A little cloudy on formatting that list of lab results, vital signs, or other phrases? Check the list of commonly dictated phrases and how to transcribe them in Appendix B. Appendix C is dedicated to those perennial favorites: full-length sample transcribed reports.

Appendix A

Glossary

· ·

1099-K: A recently added federal tax form used to report payments made via third-party payment processors. Copies are sent to the Internal Revenue Service and the recipient of the income. A medical transcriptionist working as an independent contractor may receive this form instead of a 1099-MISC if the client pays via a third-party system like PayPal instead of directly.

1099-MISC: A federal tax form used to report certain types of payments made, including amounts paid to independent contractors. Copies are sent to the Internal Revenue Service and the recipient of the income. Medical transcriptionists working as independent contractors frequently receive these.

AAMT: *See* American Association for Medical Transcription.

ABCZ system: A widely used system for creating shortcuts that are easy to remember for use in word expanders. The central rule in the system is to use the first three letters and last letter of a word. Thus, the shortcut for the word *absolutely* is "absy."

account specifics: Transcription rules that pertain to a particular client account. They may deviate from industry standard transcription guidelines.

accredited: A program or organization that has been assessed and found to meet a predetermined set of requirements and quality standards set by the accrediting body. Medical facilities, educational organizations, and training programs are common examples of entities that purse accreditation.

ACE: Annual Convention and Exposition of the Association for Healthcare Documentation Integrity (AHDI) industry association. This is the premier conference for medical transcriptionists.

acute care transcription: Transcription performed for facilities (usually hospitals) that provide emergency services and short-term medical care for immediate and urgent illnesses and injuries.

AHDI: *See* Association for Healthcare Documentation Integrity.

AHIMA: *See* American Health Information Management Association.

allied health profession: A profession that is outside the medical, dental, optometric, podiatric, and pharmaceutical fields but provides related services to support them. Medical transcription often is included under this umbrella.

American Association for Medical Transcription (AAMT): The former name of the Association for Healthcare Documentation Integrity (AHDI).

American Health Information Management Association (AHIMA): A professional association for the field of medical records management.

American Medical Informatics Association (AMIA): A professional association for the field of health and biomedical informatics.

American Recovery and Reinvestment Act of 2009 (ARRA): Enacted in February 2009, this act, known as the "stimulus," includes the HITECH Act, which made substantial changes to healthcare-related regulations, including rules pertaining to protecting patient health information.

AMIA: *See* American Medical Informatics Association.

Arabic numeral: One of the symbols 1, 2, 3, 4, 5, 6, 7, 8, 9, or 0.

ARRA: *See* American Recovery and Reinvestment Act of 2009.

ASR: Automatic speech recognition. *See* speech recognition.

Association for Healthcare Documentation Integrity (AHDI): The leading professional association that medical transcriptionists belong to. Formerly known as the American Association for Medical Transcription (AAMT).

AutoCorrect: A feature in Microsoft Word that automatically replaces text as you type. It's often used to correct typos. It also can be used to create shortcuts (for example, *tpia* becomes "the patient is a"), but word expanders are much better for that.

AutoText: A feature in Microsoft Word for storing reusable blocks of text and/or graphics so they can be inserted into a document. AutoText can hold much longer blocks of text than AutoCorrect but doesn't insert them on the fly while you're typing.

back-end speech recognition: A speech recognition system where a recorded dictation is submitted to a central server, where it is then converted to text.

backlog: An accumulation of transcription work that has not been completed.

bandwidth: The maximum amount of data that can be sent over a network or Internet connection in a given period of time. It's kind of like the diameter of a hose: The bigger it is, the more you can send through it at once.

Big Four: A set of four reports that form the core of medical transcription work. They include history and physical examination (H&P), consultation, operative report, and discharge summary. Also called the _Basic Four._

blank: To leave an empty spot in a transcribed dictation as a placeholder for a word or phrase that couldn't be clearly determined. Blanking is often accomplished by inserting underscore characters like this: ____. _See also_ flagging.

BOS: _The Book of Style for Medical Transcription,_ published by the Association for Healthcare Documentation Integrity (AHDI).

brand name: The proprietary (and usually trademarked) name given to a drug or a product by its manufacturer. The brand name is always capitalized when transcribed. Also called a _trade name._

broadband: A high-speed Internet connection with large capacity (high bandwidth). Digital subscriber line (DSL) and cable are examples of broadband Internet connections. Satellite Internet connections are also considered broadband, but they're substantially slower than the other two.

brownout: A power fluctuation where electricity flow is temporarily reduced but not cut out entirely. This can cause lights to flicker and damage electronics, including computers. Brownouts can last from a few seconds to a few hours. They are common and can occur from something as simple as an air-conditioning unit kicking on in your home. They also can be caused by an outside source. An uninterruptable power system (UPS) is the best way to protect yourself from computer damage or loss of data due to a brownout.

business associate: A person or organization that performs services or functions for a business that involves the use or disclosure of protected health information (PHI). HIPAA laws require business associate agreements to include assurances that the associate and its subcontractors (including medical transcriptionists) will use appropriate safeguards to prevent use or disclosure of PHI.

C-Phone: A combination telephone/transcriber device made by Dictaphone Corporation that's used to access dictation stored at another location. This is usually done over a standard phone line dedicated to just this purpose. A headset and foot pedal plug into the C-Phone.

carpal tunnel syndrome (CTS): A painful condition of the hands and fingers that results from compression of the median nerve in the wrist. Commonly associated with extensive typing.

CDA: *See* clinical document architecture.

CEC: *See* CEU.

CEU: Continuing education unit, a measure used to assign value to continuing education activities. To maintain a certification, an individual often has to complete a set number of CEUs in a certain timeframe. Also called called continuing education credit (CEC) or professional development unit (PDU).

Certified Medical Transcriptionist (CMT): A professional certification that can be earned by experienced medical transcriptionists, not to be confused with certificates earned for completing medical transcription training. Only available through the Association for Healthcare Documentation Integrity (AHDI).

character count: The number of characters that constitute a line when calculating lines transcribed in a report (and thus the medical transcriptionist's pay). There is no universal standard, although 65 is common. It's critical to ask potential employers for this number and which keystrokes are counted as characters; for example, some count spaces, others don't. *See also* visual black character (VBC).

clinic transcription: Transcribing reports for physician practices and specialty clinics. This type of transcription is usually less complex than acute care (hospital) transcription, with fewer report types and a smaller knowledge pool to master.

clinical document architecture (CDA): A standardized structure for clinical documents, such as discharge summaries and progress notes, to facilitate patient documentation information exchange. This is an important component of electronic health record (EHR) technology.

CMT: *See* Certified Medical Transcriptionist.

CPL rate: Cents per line paid for each line transcribed.

CPT code: *See* current procedural terminology code.

CSR: Continuous speech recognition. *See* speech recognition.

current procedural terminology (CPT) code: A standardized numeric code used to identify a specific medical service or procedure rendered by a healthcare provider. Used for billing purposes.

DBA: Short for "doing business as." The operating name of a business, as opposed to its legal name. A medical transcriptionist who works as an independent contractor may choose to conduct business under a DBA name instead of his personal name. Also called a *fictitious business name.*

Dragon Naturally Speaking Medical: A well-known, commercially available speech recognition software marketed to medical practitioners.

E&O: *See* errors and omissions insurance.

EHR: *See* electronic health record.

electronic health record (EHR): The aggregate of all electronic medical records (EMRs) for an individual, from multiple sources. Although technically different in meaning from EMR, the terms often are used interchangeably.

electronic medical record (EMR): An electronic collection of health information on an individual created and managed by an organization; essentially the electronic equivalent of a paper medical chart.

EMR: See electronic medical record.

eponym: A word that is derived from the name of a person or place. For example, the Foley catheter was designed by Frederic Foley.

ergonomics: The study of designing equipment and processes to fit the human body with the goal of improving health, safety, and productivity.

errors and omissions (E&O) insurance: A form of business liability insurance sometimes carried by self-employed individuals.

ESL: English as a second language. ESL dictators typically have a heavy foreign accent and are more likely to commit grammatical errors.

estimated tax payments: Payments to a taxing authority based on an estimate of taxes actually owed. Must be submitted quarterly by people not subject to paycheck withholding, such as medical transcriptionists who work as independent contractors.

FICA: Social Security and Medicare taxes collected under the authority of the Federal Insurance Contributions Act (FICA). Also called *payroll taxes.*

fictitious business name: *See* DBA.

flagging: Marking parts of a transcribed dictation for further attention. This can be done to indicate suspected dictation errors or undecipherable phrases.

freelancer: A person who is self-employed. *See also* independent contractor.

front-end speech recognition: A speech recognition system where a text transcription is created in real time as a report is dictated. This allows the dictator to potentially spot and correct errors as they occur.

FTP: File transmission protocol. A computer protocol used for transmitting files. Medical transcriptionists may use an FTP program to download dictation files and upload transcribed reports.

fuzzy search: A search algorithm that returns results that are close matches for the search term, as well as results that are exact matches.

generic name: The nonproprietary and non-trademarked name of a drug.

health information management (HIM): The practice of managing healthcare data and information resources. It encompasses services related to planning, collecting, aggregating, analyzing, and disseminating individual and aggregated patient data.

health information technology (HIT): The design, development, implementation, and administration of health information across computerized systems.

Health Insurance Portability and Accountability Act of 1996 (HIPAA): This is the legislation that includes the Privacy Rule addressing the security and privacy of health data. It also requires establishment of national standards for electronic health records and addresses continuation of healthcare coverage after employment changes. All medical transcriptionists need to be familiar with this. Also known as *Public Law 104-191.*

HIM: *See* health information management.

HIPAA: *See* Health Insurance Portability and Accountability Act.

HIT: *See* health information technology.

HITECH Act: Health Information Technology for Economic and Clinical Health Act, enacted in 2009 to stimulate the adoption of electronic health records (EHRs) and health information technology (HIT). This included substantial changes to existing Health Insurance Portability and Accountability Act (HIPAA) regulations and other areas that affect medical transcriptionists.

home office deduction: An income tax deduction that is available to individuals who dedicate part of a home to business use.

homophones: Words that sound the same but differ in meaning (for example, *mucus* and *mucous*).

ICD-9: *See* International Classification of Diseases code.

ICD-10: *See* International Classification of Diseases code.

International Classification of Diseases (ICD) code: A standardized code used to identify a specific medical condition or disease a patient is being treated for. Used for billing purposes. ICD-9 is the ninth edition, which contains about 17,000 codes. ICD-10, which includes more than 150,000 codes, is being phased in. ICD-11 is under development.

independent contractor (IC): A person or business that provides services to other businesses. Many medical transcriptionists work as ICs.

informatics: The study of the use of technology resources and methods for the collection and utilization of information. Health informatics focuses on data capture, retrieval, and usage of information related to healthcare documentation and delivery.

Instant Text (IT): A word expander program widely used by medical transcriptionists.

JCAHO: *See* Joint Commission.

Joint Commission: An independent nonprofit organization that accredits and certifies hospitals and healthcare organizations that meet certain performance and quality standards. Formerly named Joint Commission on Accreditation of Hospital Organizations (JCAHO).

knowledge worker: Someone whose role is to create, modify, and synthesize information in a specific subject area rather than produce goods or services.

LPH: Average lines per hour produced by a transcriptionist. Used to track productivity.

macro: A keystroke combination or shortcut that executes a series of actions. For example, you could create a macro that copies an admitting diagnoses list, pastes it into the document, and changes the heading to "Final Diagnoses."

medical scribe: Someone who documents clinical patient encounters as they occur. The scribe works alongside the practitioner. While the provider focuses on the patient, the scribe focuses on creating the documentation by recording information.

medical spellchecker: A spellchecker that specifically includes medical terms that standard spellcheckers identify as incorrectly spelled.

medicolegal document: A document that pertains to both medicine and law (for example, consent for operation or independent medical evaluation).

MLS: Medical language specialist. Alternative title for medical transcriptionist.

MTIA: Medical Transcription Industry Alliance. This organization is no longer active, but was for 20 years and is still frequently referenced. From 2010 to 2012, it went by the name Clinical Documentation Industry Association (CDIA).

MTSO: Medical transcription service organization or medical transcription service owner. MTSOs provide transcription services to client companies.

nationals: Large transcription companies that contract with clients nationwide and employ multiple home-based transcriptionists.

OCR: *See* Office of Civil Rights.

Office of Civil Rights (OCR): The section of the U.S. Department of Health and Human Services that is charged with implementing the HITECH Act.

on hold: A transcribed report that will not be released for return to the client until further action, such as a quality review, is taken on it. Work from newly hired medical transcriptionists is often placed on hold for quality verification.

normals: Standard wording or blocks of text a dictator always uses when dictating particular reports. A dictator may say "insert my normal for *x* with the following changes" instead of re-dictating it.

ordinal number: A number indicating position or order, such as first (1st), second (2nd), and third (3rd).

PDR: *Physicians' Desk Reference,* a comprehensive and often referred to reference of drug names, dosages, and related information.

PDU: Professional development unit. *See* CEU.

personal health record (PHR): A collection of personal health data and information that is maintained by the patient. This is different from EHR, which consists of data collected by institutions (such as care providers).

PHI: *See* protected health information.

PHR: *See* personal health record.

platform: *See* transcription platform.

Privacy Rule: A key part of the HIPAA act that defines a set of national standards for the protection and disclosure of individual health information (protected health information). It's officially named Standards for Privacy of Individually Identifiable Health Information, but everyone calls it "the Privacy Rule."

Protected health information (PHI): Health information that is specifically protected from disclosure under the HIPAA Privacy Rule. It is essentially any health data that can be linked to a specific individual, with a few exceptions.

PTO: Paid time off.

QA: Quality assurance. A systematic process put in place to ensure that quality requirements are fulfilled.

QA score: *See* quality score.

QR: Quality review. The process of checking transcribed work for accuracy.

quality score: An accuracy rate (for example, 98 percent) assigned to a medical transcriptionist based on the results of formal auditing of completed work.

Registered Medical Transcriptionist (RMT): A credential for entry-level medical transcriptionists that is offered by the Association for Healthcare Documentation Integrity (AHDI).

RMT: *See* Registered Medical Transcriptionist.

RSI: Repetitive strain injury. RSIs are linked to performing the same motion repeatedly over a prolonged period, such as occurs with computer work. RSIs often can be alleviated or avoided through applying ergonomic design principles.

S/L: Sounds like.

Schedule C: A federal income tax form used to report profit or loss from a business (for example, medical transcriptionist self-employment income).

scribe: *See* medical scribe

self-employment tax: Tax paid by self-employed individuals to cover Social Security and Medicare contributions (FICA) usually made by employers.

shortcut software: *See* word expander.

Shorthand: A word expander program widely used by medical transcriptionists.

sole proprietorship: A business owned and operated by one person.

speech recognition editing (SRE): The process of reviewing text documents that were produced using speech recognition technology in combination with the original voice file and correcting the errors they contain.

speech recognition technology (SRT): Computer software and hardware systems used to convert spoken words into text.

SpeedType: A word expander program used by medical transcriptionists.

SR: *See* speech recognition.

SRE: *See* speech recognition editing.

SRT: *See* speech recognition technology.

STAT: Immediately.

statutory employee: An independent contractor (IC) who is treated as an employee for particular tax purposes. For a statutory employee, the company pays half the worker's FICA (Social Security and Medicare) tax and withholds the other half through paycheck withholding. A regular IC pays both halves herself in the form of self-employment tax.

SUM program: A medical transcription training curriculum created by Health Professions Institute (HPI). Part or all of it is incorporated into many MT training programs, especially the SUM practice dictations component.

TAT: Turnaround time. Elapsed time between completion of a dictation and when it's delivered in transcribed form.

tax deduction: A deduction from gross income that results in a lower taxable income (it lowers the amount you actually pay tax on).

template: A starting point for transcribing a report that includes standard headings and formatting used in that type of report.

transcription log: A record of transcription reports completed and when they were done.

transcription platform: A system used for managing transcription and, in some cases, associated workflow. Examples include DocQScribe, Emdat, and Microsoft Word.

UPS: Uninterruptible power supply. A battery-powered device you can plug your computer into that allows it to keep running in case of power failure or voltage fluctuations.

USB: Universal serial bus. A connection technology for attaching external devices, such as a foot pedal or headphones, to a computer.

verbatim transcription: A transcription of exactly what the dictator said, without grammatical errors corrected or any other changes made.

visual black character (VBC): Any printed letter, number, symbol, or punctuation mark visible to the naked eye when viewing a document. Excludes spaces, blank lines and hidden formatting. Sometimes applied when defining how many characters are considered a line.

voice recognition (VR): Identification of a voice pattern as belonging to a particular individual. Technically different in meaning from speech recognition, but often used interchangeably.

WAV pedal: A foot pedal that plugs into your computer and is used to control dictation playback, including rewind, fast-forward, and play.

withholding: Money deducted from a paycheck total by the payer, before sending the payment to the recipient, usually for the purpose of paying taxes.

word expander: Software that automatically expands abbreviations and previously defined shortcuts into full text as you type. A top productivity tool used by medical transcriptionists. Examples include Instant Text, Shorthand, and SpeedType.

Appendix B

Commonly Dictated Phrases and How to Transcribe Them

· ·

*R*eferences and examples are two of a medical transcriptionist's best friends. In this chapter, you get a bit of both. The examples demonstrate how to transcribe phrases you'll routinely encounter while transcribing:

- ✔ Laboratory tests
- ✔ Medically necessary units of measure
- ✔ Medications
- ✔ Physical examinations

Then you dip into examples from two areas that are both specialties and routine: our hearts and childbirth.

Transcribing Lab Data

Laboratory tests are like herds of elephants: The same ones hang around together all the time. A key to correctly transcribing lab data is to know which herds each test travels with. Then simply separate tests with commas and herds by periods. In the following example, the first three values belong to the blood cell herd, and the next four are electrolytes:

> **Dictated:** WBC count 8.2 hemoglobin 10.4 hematocrit 37 sodium 141 potassium 6.2 chloride 103 CO2 26

> **Transcribed:** WBC count 8.2, hemoglobin 10.4, hematocrit 37. Sodium 141, potassium 6.2, chloride 103, CO2 of 26

TIP

CO2 26 becomes CO2 of 26 to avoid potential confusion caused by putting the numbers directly beside each other. Also, note the period between hematocrit and sodium — that's where the new test group begins.

Table B-1 lists common laboratory herds (that is, profiles and panels) and the tests they include. Study up, because there's a more complex example ahead. Note that this isn't a comprehensive list. It includes the tests you'll encounter most often. The bits in parentheses are alternate names for the preceding terms.

Table B-1	Lab Test Groups
Test Group	*Includes Some or All Of . . .*
BMP (basic metabolic panel, blood chemistry)	sodium (Na), potassium (K), chloride (Cl), bicarbonate (bicarb, CO2), BUN, creatinine, glucose, calcium
CMP (comprehensive metabolic panel, chem panel)	BMP plus: albumin, total protein, ALP, ALT, AST, bilirubin
CBC (complete blood count)	RBCs, WBCs, hemoglobin (H, Hg, Hgb), hematocrit (crit, H, Hct), MCH, MCV, MCHC, platelet count
CBC with differential (diff)	CBC plus: neutrophils (polys, segs, bands), lymphocytes (lymphs), eosinophils (eos), monocytes (monos), basophils (basos), sometimes myelocytes (myelos)
ABGs (arterial blood gases, blood gasses)	pH, oxygen (O2), PO2, PCO2, oxygen saturation (O2 saturation), bicarbonate, base excess, base deficit
cardiac-related (this isn't a formal a group, but these are often together), also referred to as cardiac enzymes	troponin, troponin I, creatinine kinase (CK), CK-MB, myoglobin, lactate dehydrogenase (LDH), BNP (brain natriuretic peptide, B-type natriuretic peptide)
coagulation profile (coags, PT/INR)	PT (pro time), PTT, INR fibrin, fibrinogen, prothrombin, clotting time, factors (I, II, III, V, VII, VIII, IX, X, XI, XIII)
electrolyte panel (lytes)	sodium (Na), potassium (K), chloride (Cl), serum bicarbonate (bicarb, CO2)
LFTs (liver function tests, liver panel)	AST, ALT, alkaline phosphatase (ALP, alk phos), bilirubin (bili), albumin, total protein; less often: GGT, LDH, PT, PTT
lipid profile/panel	total cholesterol, HDL, LDL, triglycerides, VLDL
TFTs (thyroid function tests/panel)	TSH, T3, free T3, T4, free T4
UA (urinalysis)	pH, specific gravity (SG), glucose, protein, blood, bilirubin, nitrites, leukocyte esterase, ketones sediment, red blood cells, white blood cells, crystals, casts, squamous cells, bacteria

Now that you know how test grouping works, take a peek at this properly transcribed example that includes a bunch of them:

> LABORATORY DATA: Sodium 138, potassium 6.4, chloride 108, bicarbonate 18, BUN 86, creatinine 6.4, glucose 138. AST 26, ALT 20, alk phos 229, total bilirubin 0.7, albumin 3, total protein 6.9. WBC 8.2, hemoglobin 10.4, hematocrit 31, platelets 277. PT greater than 100, INR greater than 14, PTT 146.5. ABG: pH 7.19, pCO2 of 37, pO2 of 163, oxygen saturation 99% on room air. UA shows trace protein, trace glucose, moderate epithelial cells, 4 to 10 hyaline casts, 0 to 2 red blood cells, few bacteria, 2 to 5 white blood cells.

Grams Percent and Other Units of Measure

You probably know centimeters from inches, but chances are, *grams percent* isn't in your everyday vocabulary. It and other measurement terms like it have to be transcribed in very specific ways. Table B-2 lists measurements that dictators are particularly fond of and how to transcribe them.

Table B-2	Transcribing Units of Measure
Dictated	*Transcribe*
cc's (of liquid)	mL (this is done because cc is considered a dangerous abbreviation)
centimeters squared	cm^2 or sq cm NOT cm2
cubic centimeters	cm^3 or cu cm NOT cm3
cubic millimeters	mm^3 or cu mm NOT mm3
deciliter	dL
grams per deciliter	g/dL
grams percent	gm%
half percent	0.5%
hertz	Hz
international units	IU
international units per liter	IU/L
kilogram	kg

(continued)

Table B-2 *(continued)*

Dictated	Transcribe
liters	L
liters per minute	L/min
meters cubed	m^3 or cu m NOT m3
meters per second	m/s
meters squared	m^2 or sq m NOT m2
micrograms	mcg
micrograms per minute	mcg/min
milliequivalents	mEq
milligrams of mercury	mmHg
milligrams per deciliter	mg/dL
milliliters per kilogram	mL/kg
millimeters per hour	mm/h
millimoles	mmol
milliseconds	msec or ms
moles	mol
moles per liter	mol/L
nanograms per milliliter	ng/mL
ohms	ohms
per cubic millimeter	$/m^3$ or /cu mm
per high power field	/hpf
point 25 percent	0.25%
point 5 percent	0.5%
quarter percent	0.25%
volts	V

Units of measure aren't always abbreviated. Metric units, like centimeter, are always abbreviated except when not connected to a number. Nonmetric measurements, such as inches and pounds, are spelled out. For example:

Dictated: The two centimeter wound is about a centimeter below his knee.

Transcribed: The 2 cm wound is about a centimeter below his knee.

Dictated: The newborn weighs six pounds eight ounces (two thousand nine hundred forty eight grams).

Transcribed: The newborn weighs 6 pounds 8 ounces (2948 g).

Transcribing Medications

The medication list for a seriously ill patient can contain more ingredients than a Julia Child recipe does. The following examples demonstrate how to sort out the complex stew of numbers and medical lingo:

Dictated: Darvocet N one hundred one tablet p o q four to six h p r n

Transcribed: Darvocet-N 100 one tablet p.o. q.4-6 h. p.r.n.

The number *one* is spelled out because it is immediately beside another number. If it were transcribed as 100 1 tablet, it would be ripe for confusion or error. Also note the space before the *h* in *q.4-6 h.*

Dictated: potassium chloride forty milliequivalents p o q d

Transcribed: potassium chloride 40 mEq p.o. daily

q.d. is replaced with *daily* because *q.d.* is considered a dangerous abbreviation.

Dictated: clonidine point one milligram p o b i d

Transcribed: clonidine 0.1 mg p.o. b.i.d.

Note the zero added before .1 and the space between *p.o.* and *b.i.d.*

Don't know your *b.i.d.* from your *p.r.n.?* Consider putting yourself through the medical language boot camp in Chapter 5.

Commonly Dictated Physical Exam Phrases

Many medical reports include a complete or limited physical exam (PE). Table B-3 lists phrases commonly dictated in specific PE exam sections.

Table B-3   Commonly Dictated Physical Exam Phrases

Physical Exam Section	Commonly Dictated Phrases
Vital Signs	Temperature 98.7, pulse 92, blood pressure 130/88, respirations 18. O2 saturation 98% on room air.
General	patient is an x-year-old well-developed, well-nourished male/female
	patient is well developed and well nourished (**Note:** No hyphens in this form)
	awake, alert, and oriented x3 (times 3), in no acute distress, resting comfortably, pleasant and cooperative.
HEENT (head, eyes, ears, nose, throat)	Head: Normocephalic, atraumatic.
	Eyes: PERRLA, EOMI. No nystagmus. Conjugate gaze. Pupils equal, round, reactive to light and accommodation. Extraocular movements are intact. Pink conjunctivae, anicteric sclerae. No scleral icterus. Visual fields full.
	Ears: TMs clear bilaterally. TMs pearly gray.
	Nose and throat: Moist mucous membranes. Oral mucosa moist. Oropharynx is clear. Oropharynx without erythema or exudate.
	Mouth: No lesions. Edentulous. Poor dentition.
Neck	Supple. No lymphadenopathy. No bruit. No JVD or thyromegaly. Trachea midline. No jugular venous distension. No JVP elevation. Carotid pulses 2+ (two plus) bilaterally.
Breasts	No masses. No supraclavicular or axillary adenopathy. Nipples everted. No nipple discharge.
Chest	See lungs and cardiovascular headings. Chest is primarily used in place of one or both of those.
Lungs/pulmonary	Clear to auscultation bilaterally. Clear to auscultation and percussion (A and P). No rales, rhonchi, or wheezes. Good air entry bilaterally. No accessory muscle use.
	Diminished breath sounds. Coarse breath sounds. Decreased breath sounds in lower lung fields. Audible expiratory wheezing. Crackles at the bases. Prolonged expiratory phase. Scattered rhonchi and wheezes.

Physical Exam Section	Commonly Dictated Phrases
Heart/cardiovascular/ cor	Regular rate and rhythm. Regular S1, S2. No S3. No S4. No murmur, rub, or gallop. Normal PMI. PMI non-displaced. First and second heart sounds heard. No murmurs appreciated.
	Irregularly irregular rhythm. Grade 2/6 (two over six) systolic murmur.
Abdomen	Soft, nontender, nondistended. No organomegaly or masses. Positive bowel sounds. Normoactive bowel sounds. Scaphoid. Mildly obese. Morbidly obese. No rebound, guarding, or tenderness. No hepatomegaly or splenomegaly. No visceromegaly.
Back/spine	No CVA tenderness. Spine unremarkable.
Extremities	No clubbing, cyanosis, or edema. Peripheral pulses 2+ bilaterally. No calf tenderness
	Trace pedal edema. Bilateral pitting edema. Diminished pedal pulses.
Skin	No rashes or lesions.
Neurological/Central Nervous System (CNS)	Grossly nonfocal. Alert and oriented x3. No dysarthria or aphasia. Cranial nerves II through XII (2 through 12) intact. Deep tendon reflexes (DTRs) are symmetric. Motor and sensory normal. Tongue is midline. Plantar reflexes downgoing.

Commonly Dictated Obstetrics Phrases

You'll likely encounter obstetric (OB) phrases more often than you antici-pate. They appear in discharge summaries, clinic notes, and, of course, birth summaries. The verbal shortcuts they contain can be tricky to transcribe at first, but with a few examples at hand, you've got nothing to worry about.

A para what? Transcribing obstetric history

A woman's pregnancy and childbirth history is summarized using secret code. (actually, it's the GPA and TPAL systems explained in Chapter 14). Here are some examples on how to transcribe it:

Dictated: a 32 year old gravida three para two at forty weeks gestational age

Transcribed: a 32-year-old gravida 3 para 2 at 40 weeks' gestational age.

Note the apostrophe at the end of *weeks*. If it said "weeks of gestational age" instead, the apostrophe wouldn't be called for.

> **Dictated:** Obstetric history G two P one A one
>
> **Transcribed:** Obstetric history: G2, P1, A1.

> **Dictated:** Obstetric history three one zero four
>
> **Transcribed:** Obstetric history: 3-1-0-4.

The next example mixes the GPA and TPAL systems, a fairly common dictator habit.

> **Dictated:** a 23 year old G four P one zero two one female at term.
>
> **Transcribed:** a 23-year-old G4, P1-0-2-1 female at term.

If this *gravida, para,* and *TPAL* stuff is unfamiliar, Chapter 14 will reveal all.

Another thing OB docs love to do is cram as many prenatal labs into a single sentence as possible. Here's an example, pre-transcribed for you.

> Mother is O positive, GBS negative, hepatitis B surface antigen negative, rubella immune, RPR nonreactive, HIV negative.

Labor-in-progress reports

During childbirth, someone periodically takes a peek at the mother's private parts and gives a status update. Allegedly, it's to determine if labor is progressing, but some suspect it's really to see if the doctor has time for another round of golf. Here are some examples:

> **Dictated:** On exam she was four centimeters dilated, seventy percent effaced and minus two station
>
> **Transcribed:** On exam, she was 4 cm dilated, 70% effaced, and –2 station.

> **Dictated:** On exam she was four centimeters seventy percent minus one
>
> **Transcribed:** On exam, she was 4 cm, 70%, and –1.

Everyday Cardiology Phrases

Cardiology dictation is a special blend of acronyms, Arabic and Roman numerals, and hyphens. The examples in this section cover things you may encounter while transcribing EKG findings or the cardiovascular section of a physical exam. For more complex stuff, you'll need a specialty reference at hand.

Heart sounds and murmurs

When a physician listens to a patient's heart (called *auscultation*), one of the things she's looking for are four distinct heart sounds. The dictator may refer to them as S1, S2, S3, S4 or first, second, third, fourth. Here's an example:

Dictated: First and second heart sound heard. No S3 or S4.

Transcribed: First and second heart sound heard. No S3 or S4.

The preceding example was transcribed exactly as dictated.

Abnormal heart sounds, or *murmurs,* are dictated and transcribed as one number "over" another, like this:

Dictated: Grade two over six systolic murmur.

Transcribed: Grade 2/6 systolic murmur.

Dictated: Grade two to three over four murmur.

Transcribed: Grade 2 to 3 over 4 murmur OR Grade 2/4 to 3/4 murmur.

The bottom number always will be 6 or 4.

Transcribing EKG findings

EKGs can be done in a physician's office, emergency room, specialty clinic, and quite possibly on the kitchen table. To transcribe one, it helps to have a little background knowledge.

An EKG records electrical activity of the heart. A bunch of wires are attached to the patient, and the recording begins. Each wire in the bunch is called a *lead,* and each lead has a special name that involves a Roman numeral. The resulting recording is a graph that shows electrical activity in the form of waves. Someone reads it, dictates the results, and you transcribe it, like this:

> A 12-lead EKG shows normal sinus rhythm. No ST abnormality. QTC is prolonged at 497 msec. Nonspecific T-wave flattening in leads III and aVF.

Got it? If so, congrats! If not, rest assured, you are not alone. Knowing where to put hyphens and what to capitalize and not, is challenging. The following list of properly punctuated EKG phrases should help:

first-degree AV block

right bundle branch block

poor R-wave progression.

precordial leads (not precardial or pericardial)

nonspecific ST changes

no ST-T changes

ST-segment depression

no acute ST elevations

right axis deviation

Q waves in lead III

normal PR, QRS, and QT intervals

prolonged PR interval

inverted T waves in leads I, aVL, V1, V2, and V3.

no evidence of ischemia

non-Q-wave myocardial infarction

A hyphen only goes between a letter and the word *wave* (T-wave) if the term is used as an adjective (for example, *T-wave inversions* but *inverted T waves*). The only EKG leads that start with a lowercase letter are *aVF, aVR,* and *aVL.*

Appendix C

Sample Reports

• •

*W*ith two exceptions, the sample reports in this appendix stick to the formatting styles recommended in *The Book of Style for Medical Transcription,* 3rd Edition, by AHDI (see Chapter 6). There are deviants in every crowd, and in this chapter they're the operative report and the independent medical evaluation (IME). The operative report demonstrates the common practice of starting text on the same line as the heading rather than beneath it, which allows more stuff to fit on a page. IMEs are as much legal opinions as medical reports, so they're excused from doing what the BOS says.

History and Physical Examination

CHIEF COMPLAINT

Shortness of breath.

HISTORY OF PRESENT ILLNESS

This is a 56-year-old woman with past medical history of diabetes, CAD, hypertension, and dyslipidemia who came to the emergency room with a chief complaint of cough, shortness of breath, and chest congestion for the last month associated with generalized weakness, feeling dizzy, and no appetite. In emergency room, patient's saturation was found to be 88% on 2 L of nasal cannula. Patient was subsequently admitted to the hospital for further observation and management.

PAST MEDICAL HISTORY

Diabetes, CAD, hypertension, and dyslipidemia.

PAST SURGICAL HISTORY

C-sections x2, laparoscopic laparotomy for lysis of adhesions.

FAMILY HISTORY

Positive for CVA that runs in the family. No history of diabetes or cancer in the family.

SOCIAL HISTORY

Patient is currently unemployed. Quit smoking 5½ years ago. Denies alcohol or drug abuse.

ALLERGIES

ALLERGIC TO PENICILLIN.

HOME MEDICATIONS

1. Zocor 40 mg p.o. nightly.

2. Novolog 70/30, 65 units subcu nightly.

3. Atenolol 75 mg p.o. daily.

4. Aspirin 81 mg p.o. daily.

REVIEW OF SYSTEMS

As above. Otherwise negative all 12 points.

PHYSICAL EXAMINIATION

General: In no acute distress.

Vital signs: On admission, blood pressure 149/70, heart rate 56, respiratory rate 22, oxygen saturation 91% on nasal cannula, temperature 96.6.

HEENT: Normocephalic, atraumatic.

Neck: Supple. No JVD. No thyromegaly appreciated.

Lungs: Decreased breath sounds bilaterally. Wheezing bilaterally.

Cardiovascular: S1, S2. Regular. No murmur appreciated.

Abdomen: Bowel sounds present. Soft, nontender. No organomegaly appreciated.

Extremities: No edema bilaterally. No calf tenderness bilaterally.

Neurologic: Awake, alert, oriented x3. Grossly nonfocal.

LABORATORY DATA

On admission was significant for potassium 2.8. Glucose 177. BNP 215. White count 7.1, hemoglobin 14.1.

RADIOLOGY

Chest x-ray: Mild pulmonary vascular congestion without evidence of congestive heart failure. No active infiltrates noted.

ASSESSMENT

1. Dyspnea, the cause to be determined.

2. Diabetes.

3. Coronary artery disease (CAD).

4. Hypertension.

5. Dyslipidemia.

6. Fatigue.

PLAN

Patient was admitted to medical floor for further treatment. She has been treated with IV antibiotics, IV Solu-Medrol, and DuoNeb. Blood cultures, sputum culture, urinalysis ordered in emergency room. We will follow the results. We will obtain 2D echo to evaluate ejection fraction (EF), left ventricle function. We will monitor patient's oxygenation. We will supplement electrolytes. We will monitor patient closely.

Consultation Report

REASON FOR CONSULTATION: Left shoulder tendinitis.

HISTORY OF PRESENT ILLNESS: Dr. Algood refers this 47-year-old general manager of an auto body shop for consultation and opinion regarding left shoulder pain. She has had pain for about a year. She does not remember any moment of injury. She is an active tennis player and hiker and lifts weights. She has pain mostly in the evenings. It is anterior and can radiate into the humerus. She feels her strength is okay. She reports no clicking, popping, numbness, or tingling. She has no symptoms in her right shoulder.

PAST MEDICAL HISTORY: Left knee meniscus repair in 2002.

ALLERGIES: None.

FAMILY HISTORY: History of arthritis in mother.

SOCIAL HISTORY: She is married with 2 children. Nonsmoker, occasional alcohol.

PHYSICAL EXAMINATION: On exam, she is a fit-appearing woman 5 feet 5 inches tall and weighing 145 pounds. Her left shoulder has no atrophy. There is no tenderness over the AC joint or biceps. She has full flexion with a negative impingement test and abduction. She lacks about 10 degrees of external rotation, has full internal rotation but with mild pain. She had slight crepitus on passive motion, a negative apprehension test, and good strength on resisted testing.

IMAGING: X-rays of the shoulder reveal calcification in the soft tissues over the greater tuberosity. Glenohumeral joint and AC joint look good. Normal interval between the humeral head and the acromion.

IMPRESSION: Left calcific rotator tendinitis.

PLAN: I have referred her to Winston PT for a shoulder rehab program. Cautioned her about overusing it. Will plan to see her back in 5 to 6 weeks.

(DICTATED BUT NOT READ)

Consultation Letter

RE: O'Skar, Brady

DOB: 7/3/1930

Dear Dr. McGovern:

I saw Mr. O'Skar today. As you know, he is a 79-year-old male with obesity, hypertension, osteoarthritis, chronic renal insufficiency with a creatinine of 1.8, who is scheduled for hip replacement in 1–2 months.

His current medications are Avapro 300 mg daily, atenolol 25 mg daily, Lasix 20–40 mg daily, Triam/HCT 75/25 once a day, and diclofenac 50 mg t.i.d. p.r.n. He has no known drug allergies.

Brady's medical history is notable for no history of heart disease, heart failure, diabetes, or lung disease. He does have some mild renal insufficiency; again, creatinine 1.8 with a repeat pending. He has had occasional bradycardia on exam with rates into the 40s. He has had no symptoms of hypotension, etc.

On exam today his weight was 285 pounds. His BP was 143/72. His heart rate was 57 and regular. His lungs were clear. Heart sounds regular. Abdomen obese. EKG showed a heart rate of 57 and a 1st degree AV block; otherwise normal EKG.

I think he is at low risk for any medical complications perioperatively. If bradycardia is an issue, the atenolol could always be decreased or held. I have told him to continue his Avapro, atenolol, and diuretic daily. Again, the diuretic could be held preoperatively. I do not think his renal situation should be a significant factor, but repeat lab work is pending.

Thank you for this consultation.

Sincerely,

Kenneth Hamilton, MD

Discharge Summary

DISCHARGE DIAGNOSIS

Colitis, most likely viral etiology, resolved.

REASON FOR ADMISSION

Please see admission history and physical for detailed information.

LABORATORY DATA

WBC 5.2, hemoglobin 12.2, hematocrit 40.1, platelets 212,000. Sodium 136, potassium 3.7, chloride 101, bicarb 26. Liver function tests within normal limits.

IMAGING

CT of the abdomen on admission showed a long region of mural thickening involving the transverse colon, most consistent with colitis.

CONSULTATION

Gastroenterology.

HOSPITAL COURSE

This is a 27-year-old gentleman with no significant past medical history presenting with abdominal pain. The patient initially received IV fluids. Stool studies were ordered, and the patient was started on Flagyl 500 mg q.8 h. The patient also received IV Dilaudid. Currently he is pain free, and his stool studies are pending. Gastroenterology was consulted. They recommended to advance his diet, and he tolerated his diet very well. We discontinued his Flagyl. On the day of discharge, he is clinically and hemodynamically stable.

PHYSICAL EXAMINATION

Vital signs: Temperature 98.8, heart rate 88, respiratory rate 18, blood pressure 117/68. Alert and oriented x3. HEENT: Pupils are equally reactive to light and accommodation. Extraocular movements are intact. Neck supple, no JVD, no lymphadenopathy. Cardiovascular system: S1, S2 present. No murmur. Respiratory system: Clear lung sounds. No wheeze or crackles. Abdomen: Soft, nontender. Bowel sounds present. Extremities: No pedal edema. Central nervous system: No focal neurological deficits.

CONDITION ON DISCHARGE

Stable.

DISPOSITION

Discharge to home.

DISCHARGE MEDICATION

Percocet 1 or 2 tablets p.o. q.4-6 h. p.r.n. pain.

DISCHARGE INSTRUCTIONS

Follow up with the gastroenterology clinic in 2 weeks.

Time spent: More than 45 minutes.

Death Summary

DATE OF ADMISSION: 00/00/0000

DATE OF DEATH: 00/00/0000

HOSPITAL COURSE

This gentleman suffered from interstitial lung disease as well as metastatic carcinoma of the lungs. He was admitted with metastatic and compressive spinal cord disease. He went on to suffer from degeneration of that problem. Possible surgical options were absolutely impossible and insurmountable, technically speaking. The patient was DNR and became care and comfort. He went on to pass away peacefully.

CAUSE OF DEATH

End of life due to terminal lung carcinoma in a setting of end-stage renal disease, clinical COPD from a lifetime of smoking, and being DNR/DNI. The patient was pronounced dead on January 11, 2012, at 9:54 p.m.

Operative Report

PREOPERATIVE DIAGNOSIS: Right medial meniscus tear.

POSTOPERATIVE DIAGNOSIS: Right lateral meniscus tear.

OPERATION: Right partial lateral meniscectomy.

ANESTHESIA: General.

ESTIMATED BLOOD LOSS: Minimal.

TOURNIQUET TIME: None.

COMPLICATIONS: None.

DISPOSITION: The patient was taken to the recovery room in good condition.

INDICATIONS FOR PROCEDURE: The patient is a 37-year-old female who injured her knee while playing hockey approximately 4 months ago. She continued to have pain despite exercise and anti-inflammatories, thus indicating the need for arthroscopy.

PROCEDURE: After suitable anesthesia was achieved, the patient's knee was injected with 30 mL of 0.25% Marcaine with epinephrine. Her knee was sterilely prepped and draped in standard orthopedic fashion. A superomedial portal was established and inflow established through this portal. An anterolateral portal was then made and the arthroscope inserted. The knee was comprehensively examined. All compartments were examined, and the medial compartment, including meniscus and articular surface actually looked very good. The meniscus was probed, and there were no tears seen or palpated although the meniscus did seem to have a little bit of flounce to it. The anterior cruciate ligament was probed and was intact. The lateral compartment did reveal a complex tear at the junction of the anterior horn and middle third of the meniscus, and this was trimmed using a combination of basket forceps and full radius synovial resector until the meniscus was stable. Some mild synovitis in the lateral compartment and gutter was debrided using the full radius synovial resector. The patellofemoral joint and all compartments were once again comprehensively examined, and no further pathology was noted. The knee was thoroughly lavaged. A sterile dressing was applied. The patient was awakened and taken to the recovery room in good condition.

Procedure Note

PROCEDURE

All-night diagnostic polysomnography.

INDICATIONS FOR PROCEDURE

The patient has the symptoms of loud snoring and daytime sleepiness. She wakes up and has trouble falling back to sleep. She frequently falls asleep while sitting quietly, like in churches, meetings, or watching TV. She has a history of high blood pressure and hypertension.

MEDICATIONS

1. Maxzide.

2. Lotensin.

SUMMARY

Total recording time was 415 minutes, out of which the patient slept for 407 minutes, achieving the sleep efficiency of 90%. Sleep onset latency was 4 minutes, and REM onset from sleep onset was 61 minutes.

Sleep architecture demonstrated that the patient spent approximately 31% of total sleep time in REM sleep, 49% in stage 2, and 20% in slow-wave sleep. The patient had 98 hypopneas, 2 mixed apneas, and 4 obstructive apneas. Her index was 36 events per hour in the REM sleep and 17 events total per hour.

Baseline oxygen saturation was 94% with a minimum oxygen desaturation down to 77%. Loud snoring was seen throughout the night. The patient spent 24% of her total sleep time snoring.

A few leg movements were seen, and spontaneous arousals were seen, with an arousal index of approximately 10 arousals per hour.

IMPRESSION

This study showed that the patient has a sleep apnea mostly seen in rapid eye movement (REM) sleep, with an index of 37 events per hour in the REM sleep and total index of 17 events per hour, with oxygen desaturation down to 77% from the baseline of 94%. Loud snoring and spontaneous arousals were also noted.

RECOMMENDATION

1. Nasal CPAP titration study.

2. Avoid alcohol and sleep medications.

3. Avoid operating machinery or driving if drowsy or sleepy.

Progress Note

SUBJECTIVE: An 82-year-old female here for a follow-up on her medical issues, which include atrial fibrillation, valvular heart disease, history of psychiatric disorder.

MEDICATIONS: Mellaril 25 mg at bedtime, Toprol 25 t.i.d., Lasix 40 daily, warfarin 5 mg as directed.

REVIEW OF SYSTEMS: She complains of left shoulder pain. She has had frozen shoulder and arthritis there since 2001. She feels it is getting worse. She denies recent falls or trauma. She has some baseline dyspnea on exertion. No PND or orthopnea. No edema.

EXAMINATION: On exam her weight is 148, BP 110/69, pulse in the 70s. Lungs clear, no wheezes or rales, good breath sounds. Left shoulder has very minimal range of motion with some pain with unassisted motion. Extremities with no edema. Heart sounds irregular with a loud systolic murmur.

ASSESSMENT/PLAN:

1. Left shoulder pain: It is certainly consistent with a frozen right shoulder. Will repeat an X-ray from 2003. She does not seem interested in PT. She can use Tylenol p.r.n. and will follow her progress.

2. Atrial fibrillation: Stable. Good rate control. Continue anticoagulation. Will follow accordingly.

3. Valve disease: Stable. Will check chemistries, CBC, and follow up in 5–6 months.

4. History of anemia: Recheck CBC.

SOAP Note

S: She presents for a hospital followup. She was hospitalized with intractable back pain, radicular symptoms down the left leg. She received IV steroids, pain medication which has helped. MRI shows significant degenerative disk disease of L3, L4, L5. She went home with a Medrol Dosepak and Percocet. She has had to take minimal Percocet since being home. She has chronic neuropathic symptoms in her legs and feet which is unchanged.

O: Alert and oriented x3. No acute distress. Neck is supple. Cardiac exam is regular, S1, S2, no murmur. Abdomen soft, nontender. Extremities with trace ankle edema. Pulses bilaterally symmetrical. DTRs are 1+ in both knees.

A: Low back pain with lumbar radiculopathy. Peripheral neuropathy.

P: Referral to physical therapy for pain control and help with gait stability and decreased risk of falls. Patient could be a candidate for epidural injections if no improvement. She still has Percocet to take for pain. Continue Lyrica. Follow up in a month.

Radiology Report

PROCEDURE

MRI of lumbar spine without contrast.

REASON FOR STUDY

Low back pain.

FINDINGS

The alignment is anatomic. There are no fractures. The conus medullaris is normal. There is no spondylolysis or spondylolisthesis. The L5-S1 disc shows early degeneration and posterior annular tear without associated disc herniation, nerve impingement, or spinal canal stenosis. There is no foraminal narrowing present.

The remaining disc levels are unremarkable.

IMPRESSION

Early degenerative disease and annular tear at L5-S1 without disc herniation or spinal canal stenosis.

Summary of Labor and Delivery

PREOPERATIVE DIAGNOSIS

A 40-week intrauterine pregnancy in active labor.

POSTOPERATIVE DIAGNOSIS

Normal spontaneous vaginal delivery.

DESCRIPTION OF PROCEDURE

This 25-year-old gravida 1, para 0 was admitted in active labor with spontaneous rupture of membranes at 1400. Vaginal exam on admission was 1, 75%, –1 station. The patient requested epidural. This was administered at 1600. With the patient pushing actively in the 2nd stage of labor, epidural anesthesia working well, fetal vertex progressed to the vaginal introitus. Nasopharynx suctioned at perineum followed by delivery of the rest of the male infant at 1840. The cord was double clamped and incised, infant given warming and drying and suctioning. Apgars noted at 9 and 9. The placenta was delivered complete, intact. Three vessels were noted in the cord. Cord blood was obtained for arterial and venous cord gas sampling. The lower genital tract was inspected. A small, midline perineal laceration was repaired with a short running suture of 2-0 chromic catgut. The uterus firmed up well. Estimated blood loss was around 300 mL. Mother and infant in good condition.

Psychiatric Assessment

CHIEF COMPLAINT

Suicidal.

HISTORY OF PRESENT ILLNESS

The patient is a 38-year-old Caucasian male with history of schizoaffective disorder, possibly bipolar disorder, has been off of medications for at least 6 months. He tells me to some extent that he has not been able to afford it because of lack of medical coverage for medications. The main reason why he checked himself in is because of suicidal thoughts. The patient further reports a roller-coaster ride in terms of his moods. He acknowledges he has bipolar disorder and needs to get back on his medications.

PAST PSYCHIATRIC HISTORY

He has been treated with a combination of Seroquel as high as 1200 mg per day and lithium 1500 mg per day. He has also been on heavy doses of Risperdal. He has been on Thorazine and BuSpar as well. His recollection of dosages is questionable.

ALCOHOL AND DRUGS

The patient has a history of very rare intake. No history of inpatient or outpatient drug or alcohol treatment problems. No DUIs, blackouts, DTs, or seizures. No history of marijuana, cocaine, heroin, PCP, LSD, or crystal methamphetamine use.

MEDICAL HISTORY

He was recently diagnosed with a sinus infection, for which he was started on Zithromax.

FAMILY PSYCHIATRIC HISTORY

No known family psychiatric history. No known family history of suicide attempts or completions. No history of drug or alcohol issues in the family.

SOCIAL HISTORY

The patient is unemployed. He does not seem to have much of a support system. He mentioned his pastor as a support system, but at the same time states that he does not want the pastor involved, because the church does not believe in him being on medications. The patient does admit to having a past history of violence, and he feels that religion is a big reason why he is able to keep himself, as well as others, safe.

MENTAL STATUS EXAMINATION

The patient is quite well groomed, clean-cut. He is alert, oriented x3, cooperative. He maintains good eye contact. There is no pressure of speech or flight of ideas, but there seems to be some religious preoccupation. His mood is euthymic. Constricted affect. No evidence of hallucinations at this time, but admits that he has had them in the past. No suicidal or homicidal ideation at this time. He seems to have partial insight and fair judgment.

DIAGNOSTIC IMPRESSION

Axis I:

Schizoaffective disorder, bipolar type.

Axis II:

Deferred.

Axis III:

Sinus infection.

Axis IV:

Poor social support.

Financial stressors.

Axis V:

Global assessment of functioning (GAF) 30.

PLAN

Patient will be admitted to the inpatient psychiatric unit. He will be restarted on lithium 300 t.i.d., Risperdal 0.5 b.i.d., and Klonopin 0.5 b.i.d. I estimate his inpatient stay will be about a week.

Independent Medical Evaluation

Re: Case, Justin

Date of Injury: November 11, 2011

Date of Examination: December 12, 2012

Introduction:

Today, at the request of Independent Examinator, LLC, I reviewed the medical records provided and completed a review on the claimant, Justin Case. History was obtained from the patient. Records were reviewed and the patient was examined in my office.

Records Reviewed:

Injury incident report, Big Box Movers records; office notes of Constance Norring, MD; Helpim Physical Therapy clinic notes; MRI imaging and reports from Seam Radiology.

History:

The patient is currently 24 years old. According to the patient, he was working as sorter for Big Box Movers. His lifting requirements were 1 to 60 pounds. On November 11, 2011, he was lifting a 50-pound box placing it to his right and on a conveyor and developed low back pain. He denied any prior back problems. He was sent home for rest and was seen in late November by his primary care doctor. He was examined. X-rays were obtained. He was given Flexeril and told to rest again. Subsequently, he had physical therapy for approximately 3 months.

He eventually saw an orthopedist who did not recommend surgery but wanted the patient to consider injection, which the patient has been reluctant to undergo.

Currently, Mr. Case continues to complain of low back pain with radiation of pain that goes to his mid-calf area. It had previously gone to his foot. He has an area of numbness on the medial aspect of the left foot. After the injury, he remained out of work until sometime in December 2011 and then returned to work for about 4 or 5 days but has been out of work since that time.

Currently, he complains of tightness in the back with minimal pain. Periodically, he has leg pain. He has developed some upper back pain. He states that motion produces pain in his back.

Physical Examination:

Examination shows a normally developed man who is ambulating without assistance. He has no limp. He has some tenderness in his low back area and his left buttock. Motion is decreased with 60 degrees of forward flexion, 10 degrees of lateral bending, and 10 degrees of extension. Strength in the lower extremities is intact. There is an area of decreased sensation over the medial aspect of the left foot. Ankle jerk on the left is markedly decreased compared to the right which is graded at 2+. Knee jerks are both 2+. The right calf measures 13¼ inches. The left calf measures 12¾ inches. There is some calf and foot pain on the left with stretch test at 80 degrees.

Diagnostic Studies:

March 3, 2012, MRI of lumbosacral spine showed an L5-S1 herniated disk, which is impinging on the S1 nerve root.

Diagnosis:

Herniated disc L5-S1, left, with localizing left leg radiculitis.

Questions and Answers to Specific Issues:

1. Has the patient reached maximum medical improvement? No. He has ongoing symptoms, although he is slowly improving. He does have clinically localized radiculitis, left leg, with clinical evidence of S1 nerve root impingement, and this is consistent with his MRI findings.

2. Is the current treatment reasonable and necessary? Yes, his current treatment is reasonable and necessary. Consideration for injection remains reasonable. Consideration for surgery may also be reasonable if he does not continue to improve.

3. If Mr. Case has not reached maximum medical improvement, based on a reasonable degree of medical certainty, when do you anticipate he will reach that point? This may be up to a year. Again, he may be a candidate for injection in his back, and surgery is not ruled out because he does have objective localizing signs.

4. Can the patient return to work with or without restrictions? If restrictions, what are they? Currently, Mr. Case is restricted from any lifting, bending, stooping, climbing, or kneeling. He may occasionally carry 5 pounds at waist level but is not allowed any lifting or bending whatsoever.

5. Is the patient able to return to work at Big Box Movers? Mr. Case has a clinically obvious herniated disc and is not likely to be able return to activities that involve lifting and bending on a permanent basis.

The above opinions are to a reasonable degree of medical certainty.

Dr. X

Index

e & Mac

2 For Dummies,
dition
-118-17679-5

e 4S For Dummies,
dition
-118-03671-6

ouch For Dummies,
dition
-118-12960-9

)S X Lion
ummies
-118-02205-4

ing & Social Media

le For Dummies
-118-08337-6

ook For Dummies,
dition
-118-09562-1

Blogging
ummies
-118-03843-7

r For Dummies,
dition
-470-76879-2

Press For Dummies,
dition
-118-07342-1

ess

Flow For Dummies
-118-01850-7

ing For Dummies,
dition
-470-90545-6

Job Searching with Social
Media For Dummies
978-0-470-93072-4

QuickBooks 2012
For Dummies
978-1-118-09120-3

Resumes For Dummies,
6th Edition
978-0-470-87361-8

Starting an Etsy Business
For Dummies
978-0-470-93067-0

Cooking & Entertaining

Cooking Basics
For Dummies, 4th Edition
978-0-470-91388-8

Wine For Dummies,
4th Edition
978-0-470-04579-4

Diet & Nutrition

Kettlebells For Dummies
978-0-470-59929-7

Nutrition For Dummies,
5th Edition
978-0-470-93231-5

Restaurant Calorie Counter
For Dummies,
2nd Edition
978-0-470-64405-8

Digital Photography

Digital SLR Cameras &
Photography For Dummies,
4th Edition
978-1-118-14489-3

Digital SLR Settings
& Shortcuts
For Dummies
978-0-470-91763-3

Photoshop Elements 10
For Dummies
978-1-118-10742-3

Gardening

Gardening Basics
For Dummies
978-0-470-03749-2

Vegetable Gardening
For Dummies,
2nd Edition
978-0-470-49870-5

Green/Sustainable

Raising Chickens
For Dummies
978-0-470-46544-8

Green Cleaning
For Dummies
978-0-470-39106-8

Health

Diabetes For Dummies,
3rd Edition
978-0-470-27086-8

Food Allergies
For Dummies
978-0-470-09584-3

Living Gluten-Free
For Dummies,
2nd Edition
978-0-470-58589-4

Hobbies

Beekeeping
For Dummies,
2nd Edition
978-0-470-43065-1

Chess For Dummies,
3rd Edition
978-1-118-01695-4

Drawing For Dummies,
2nd Edition
978-0-470-61842-4

eBay For Dummies,
7th Edition
978-1-118-09806-6

Knitting For Dummies,
2nd Edition
978-0-470-28747-7

Language & Foreign Language

English Grammar
For Dummies,
2nd Edition
978-0-470-54664-2

French For Dummies,
2nd Edition
978-1-118-00464-7

German For Dummies,
2nd Edition
978-0-470-90101-4

Spanish Essentials
For Dummies
978-0-470-63751-7

Spanish For Dummies,
2nd Edition
978-0-470-87855-2

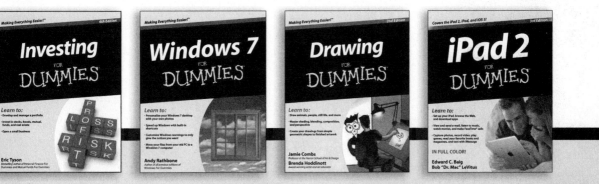

Math & Science

Algebra I For Dummies,
2nd Edition
978-0-470-55964-2

Biology For Dummies,
2nd Edition
978-0-470-59875-7

Chemistry For Dummies,
2nd Edition
978-1-1180-0730-3

Geometry For Dummies,
2nd Edition
978-0-470-08946-0

Pre-Algebra Essentials
For Dummies
978-0-470-61838-7

Microsoft Office

Excel 2010 For Dummies
978-0-470-48953-6

Office 2010 All-in-One
For Dummies
978-0-470-49748-7

Office 2011 for Mac
For Dummies
978-0-470-87869-9

Word 2010
For Dummies
978-0-470-48772-3

Music

Guitar For Dummies,
2nd Edition
978-0-7645-9904-0

Clarinet For Dummies
978-0-470-58477-4

iPod & iTunes
For Dummies,
9th Edition
978-1-118-13060-5

Pets

Cats For Dummies,
2nd Edition
978-0-7645-5275-5

Dogs All-in One
For Dummies
978-0470-52978-2

Saltwater Aquariums
For Dummies
978-0-470-06805-2

Religion & Inspiration

The Bible For Dummies
978-0-7645-5296-0

Catholicism For Dummies,
2nd Edition
978-1-118-07778-8

Spirituality For Dummies,
2nd Edition
978-0-470-19142-2

Self-Help & Relationships

Happiness For Dummies
978-0-470-28171-0

Overcoming Anxiety
For Dummies,
2nd Edition
978-0-470-57441-6

Seniors

Crosswords For Seniors
For Dummies
978-0-470-49157-7

iPad 2 For Seniors
For Dummies, 3rd Edition
978-1-118-17678-8

Laptops & Tablets
For Seniors For Dummies,
2nd Edition
978-1-118-09596-6

Smartphones & Tablets

BlackBerry For Dummies,
5th Edition
978-1-118-10035-6

Droid X2 For Dummies
978-1-118-14864-8

HTC ThunderBolt
For Dummies
978-1-118-07601-9

MOTOROLA XOOM
For Dummies
978-1-118-08835-7

Sports

Basketball For Dummies,
3rd Edition
978-1-118-07374-2

Football For Dummies,
2nd Edition
978-1-118-01261-1

Golf For Dummies,
4th Edition
978-0-470-88279-5

Test Prep

ACT For Dummies,
5th Edition
978-1-118-01259-8

ASVAB For Dummies,
3rd Edition
978-0-470-63760-9

The GRE Test For
Dummies, 7th Edition
978-0-470-00919-2

Police Officer Exam
For Dummies
978-0-470-88724-0

Series 7 Exam
For Dummies
978-0-470-09932-2

Web Development

HTML, CSS, & XHTML
For Dummies, 7th Edit
978-0-470-91659-9

Drupal For Dummies,
2nd Edition
978-1-118-08348-2

Windows 7

Windows 7
For Dummies
978-0-470-49743-2

Windows 7
For Dummies,
Book + DVD Bundle
978-0-470-52398-8

Windows 7 All-in-One
For Dummies
978-0-470-48763-1

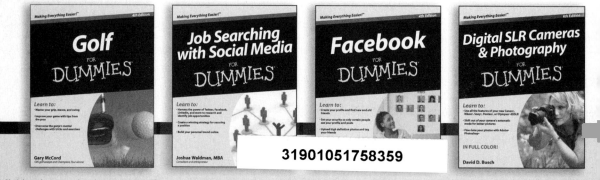